An Atlas of
PAEDIATRIC
DERMATOLOGY

Professors Carlo L. Meneghini and E. Bonifazi

Dermatological Clinic, University of Bari

Translated from the Italian and edited by

Hilary Marks and Professor Ronald Marks, FRCP, MRCPath

Foreword by
Professor Howard Maibach
Department of Dermatology, University of California

MARTIN DUNITZ

© Martin Dunitz Ltd
English language edition 1986

First published in the United Kingdom in 1986
by Martin Dunitz Ltd, The Livery House, 7-9 Pratt Street, London NW1 0AE

Reprinted 1997

British Library Cataloguing in Publication Data

Meneghini, Carlo L.
   An atlas of paediatric dermatology
   1. Paediatric dermatology
   I. Title   II. Bonifazi, E.   III. Marks, Ronald
   IV. Dermatologia pediatrica pratica. *English*
   618.92'5   RJ511

ISBN 0-906348-90-0

Printed by Kyodo Printing Industries Co Pte Ltd, Singapore

Contents

Foreword

Dr Carlo Meneghini and Dr Ernesto Bonifazi perceived an obvious and pertinent need: how to help general physicians, paediatricians, medical students and other health care professionals identify and treat the majority of the more prevalent paediatric dermatoses.

They have admirably succeeded; even an hour spent with the brief text provides practical and pertinent 'how to do it' information. The combination of concise carefully chosen descriptions and high quality photographic documentation offers a succinct and eminently workable approach not only to handling paediatric dermatology but also to grasping how it differs from the more traditional adult orientated dermatology taught to most of us.

This Atlas should rapidly increase the quality of dermatological care provided to our paediatric populations. The authors are to be congratulated for a job well done.

Howard Maibach, MD
Department of Dermatology
University of California, San Francisco

Preface

In the last thirty years there have been striking advances in paediatric dermatology. This happy state of affairs has been much helped by the co-operation of dermatologists and paediatricians. The subject has expanded vastly alongside other medical disciplines but the practical physician must still remain with his feet on the ground, in touch with day-to-day clinical problems. This consideration has guided the selection of photographs and text selected for this short commentary on skin disorders in children. It should be of assistance to all health workers who may be concerned with such patients.

The ichthyoses

This term includes a variety of disorders which are characterized by generalized scaling of the skin (the term is derived from a fanciful likeness of the scaling to fish scales). They are congenital disorders and are often due to an error of lipid metabolism (for example, steroid sulphatase deficiency in sex linked ichthyosis). The commonest form is autosomal dominant ichthyosis (ichthyosis vulgaris). This is rarely present at birth but becomes evident in the first years of life. It usually improves during the summer and worsens in cold, dry weather. Characteristically it spares the flexural areas and is accompanied by accentuation of the palmar creases. It is often said to be associated with the atopic condition, although this is not universally accepted. Xeroderma is a less severe type of disorder of keratinization with generalized roughness and dryness of the skin and keratosis pilaris (horny plugs in follicular orifices). The atopic state is often accompanied by xeroderma. Keratosis pilaris, which becomes evident in early life, can be recognized by a spiky sensation to the touch. It is mainly evident over the extensor aspects of the upper arms but when more extensive can be seen over the thighs and even over the face. Although the condition can by very persistent it tends to improve with time.

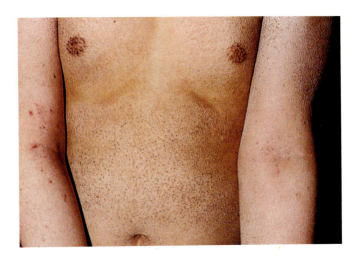

Figure 1 Ichthyosis and atopic dermatitis affecting the antecubital fossae.

Treatment Keratolytic agents such as salicylic acid (1–5 per cent) or retinoic acid in petroleum jelly (petrolatum) should be used when required temporarily to reduce the build-up of scale.

Epidermolysis bullosa

The term describes a group of congenital bullous dermatoses due to abnormalities at the dermo-epidermal junction. They are classified according to clinical and histopathological criteria. In the so-called simple forms (epidermolysis bullosa simplex) blisters form above the junctional zone in the basal layers. The dystrophic types (epidermolysis bullosa dystrophica) are characterized by the formation of bullae within or beneath the basal lamina. In the less severely affected patients blisters form mainly at sites of trauma, such as the extensor aspects of the fingers.

Figure 2 Dominant dystrophic epidermolysis bullosa with bullous lesions provoked by trauma.

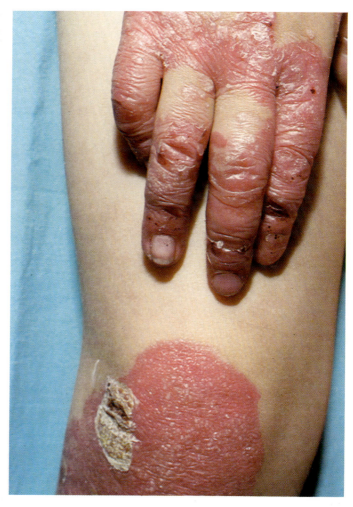

In the most disabling form (recessive dystrophic types) the bullae form independently of trauma and also involve the oral mucosa and oesophagus. These lesions may be responsible for severe deformity and functional disability and can be fatal. Blisters continue to occur but tend to be less frequent with the passage of time. Differential diagnosis may be difficult in the first few days of life when the bullous lesions must be differentiated from blisters due to a pyoderma or from rarer disorders.

Local treatment This consists of opening the bullae, the use of non-adherent dressing and application of antiseptics such as hypochlorite solution or local antimicrobiol agents.

General treatment Steroids are not usually used (although there was a vogue for high dose prednisone therapy at one time). In the recessive dystrophic form the phenytoin has been used to inhibit collagenase activity but their clinical effectiveness has not been proved. In-patient treatment may be required for the most severely affected patients.

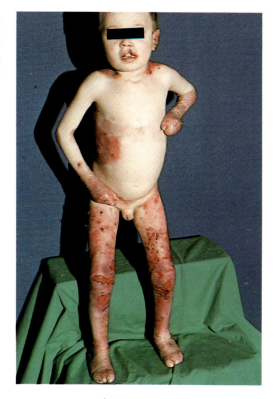

Figure 3 Recessive dystrophic epidermolysis bullosa. Bullae form on any part of the skin and may occur independently of trauma. Post-inflammatory syndactyly of the hands and feet and palatal and labial fissuring have occurred in this patient.

Congenital melanocytic naevus

The term is applied to a melanocytic naevus present at birth. The importance of these lesions is that there is a greater tendency for them to become malignant. They differ also in size – acquired naevi are rarely larger than 1 cm in diameter whereas congenital lesions are generally larger than this and may be very extensive, even covering up to 50 per cent of the body surface (cape and bathing trunk naevi – Figure 5). They differ too from acquired melanocytic naevi in that they extend more deeply into dermis and subcutaneous tissues.

Figure 4 Congenital melanocytic naevus of the lower jaw. Note the irregular distribution of pigment at the centre of the lesion.

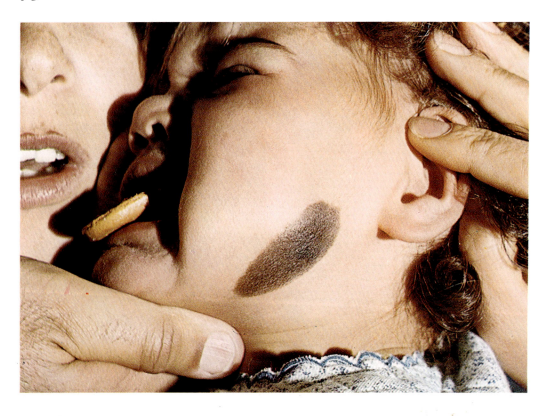

These naevi can occur on any area of the skin. They may be single isolated lesions, but are often multiple and in this case one naevus usually exceeds the size of the others. Sometimes they are slate-coloured and irregularly pigmented. While at birth they may be quite lightly pigmented, they usually darken to become quite intensely pigmented in later years. Their surface is smooth at birth but will thicken with time, eventually presenting an irregular surface. Hypertrophic hairs may often cover these lesions, leading to their designation — congenital hairy naevus – Figure 5.

Malignant melanoma may develop in these lesions as early as in the first ten years of life. This change should be suspected if a differently pigmented nodule arises in the lesions (Figure 7, 11).

Figure 5 Congenital hairy melanocytic naevus in bathing trunk distribution.

Figure 6 Congenital melanocytic naevus of the trunk.

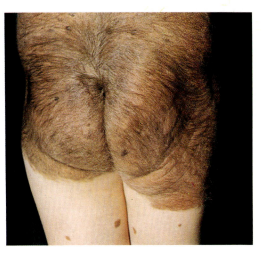

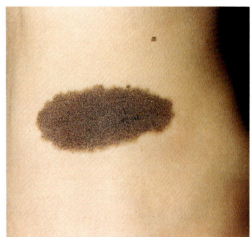

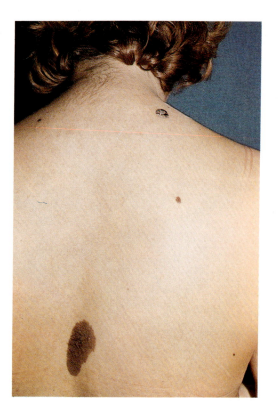

Figure 7 Multiple congenital melanocytic naevi of the trunk of a girl aged nineteen. On one of these, over the right shoulder, there is a cherry-sized nodular melanoma.

Differential diagnosis They must be distinguished from café au lait spots, Becker's naevus, naevus spilus and warty epidermal naevus. Café au lait spots are lighter in colour, always flat and smooth surfaced, and are never hairy. However, it should be remembered that von Recklinghausen's disease may occur together with congenital melanocytic naevi (Figure 11). Becker's naevus (Figure 8) is due to hypertrophy of all epidermal elements, including adnexal structures. It only becomes evident after the age of ten.

The colour of a Becker's naevus is lighter than that of a melanocytic naevus and it is always uniformly pigmented. Naevus spilus is a lightly pigmented patch surmounted by ordinary, more darkly pigmented naevi. It may have a zosterform distribution. Surgical removal is not required but it is prudent to keep it under observation (Figure 9). Epidermal naevus is

Figure 8 Becker's naevus isn't present at birth, and typically is brown and covered by thick hair.

Figure 9 Zosterform naevus spilus. On the pigmented area there are both junctional and compound naevi.

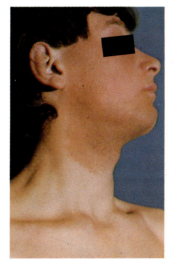
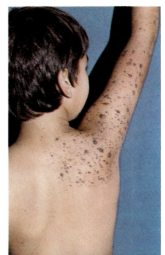

Figure 10 Warty epidermal naevus simulating melanocytic naevus. It may be differentiated by its wartiness.

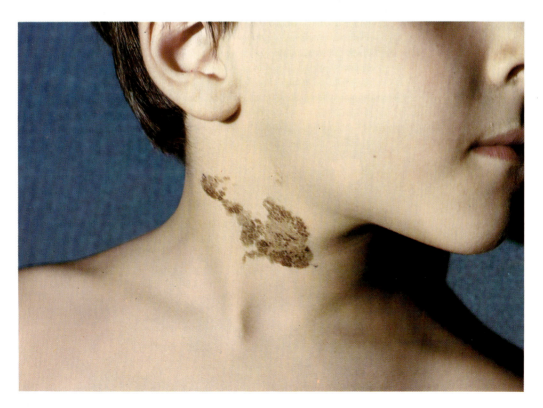

often pigmented but is usually brown rather than slate-coloured and its surface is often warty.

Treatment The treatment of congenital melanocytic naevi is controversial. Some recommend excision of such lesions as early as at three weeks old to avoid the possibility of malignant transformation later. The rationale of early removal is that naevus cell migration into the dermis is believed to occur within the first few weeks and malignant transformation may occur as early as in the first decade. The more extensive the naevus, the more the likelihood of malignant transformation and the earlier should be the surgical intervention.

However, other clinicians doubt the validity of the supposed 5 to 10 per cent rate of malignant change in these lesions and, further, doubt whether major surgery is justifiable with this degree of risk, were it to be an accurate estimate. Bilateral mastectomy isn't routinely performed on postmenopausal women who have an 8 per cent risk of carcinoma of the breast!

Our policy is to remove those lesions where the surgery involved isn't too devastating. Where very extensive lesions of the bathing trunk or cape type are involved, or where lesions occur on the face, we advise frequent clinical checks and close parental observation.

Figure 11 A nine year old girl with von Recklinghausen's neurofibromatosis and a congenital melanocytic naevus on the left side of the neck. The tumour on the naevus is a malignant schwannoma.

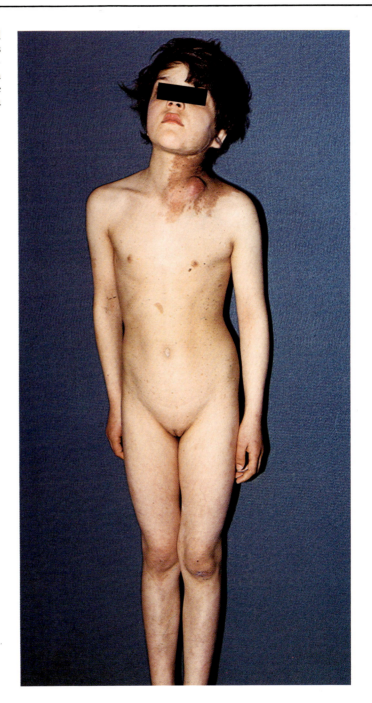

Lentigo and freckles (ephelides)

Lentigo and freckles are often confused. Freckles are a response to solar exposure in some fair-skinned individuals. They are symmetrical and more obvious in the light exposed areas, including the cheeks, the nose and over the upper part of the back and darken upon exposure to sunlight. They can be treated by inducing peeling with cardice (solid carbon dioxide sticks) or a slush of solid carbon dioxide and acetone. Lentigines are darker and smaller than freckles and are distributed at random on any body area. They represent a melanocytic naevus 'in miniature'.

In the dominantly inherited Peutz-Jeghers syndrome there is perioral and oral lentiginosis (Figure 12) and associated papillomatosis or carcinoma of the colon.

Figure 12 Perioral lentiginosis in Peutz-Jeghers syndrome.

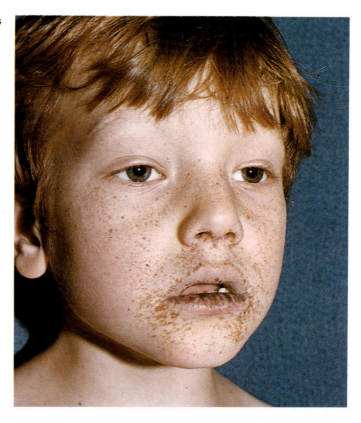

Mongolian spots

This is a naevus of dermal melanocytes occurring in almost all children of yellow and black races. It is much less frequently seen in white races. The affected area (over the sacral region) is macular and is of variable size. It is of a uniform slate grey/lead colour (Figure 13). The colour of the lesion can suggest bruising or purpura and even gluteal gangrene of the neonate. Mongolian spots tend to fade spontaneously between the ages of four and seven (Figure 14).

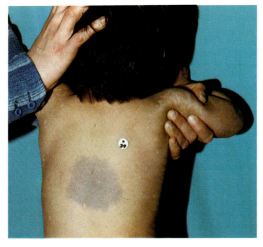

Figure 13 Mongolian spot in a Korean child at one year.

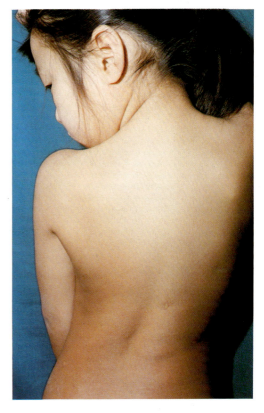

Figure 14 The same child at the age of six.

Sutton's naevus (halo naevus)

This is a cellular melanocytic naevus in which the pigment cells are destroyed and the lesion involutes spontaneously. Clinically it presents as a small protuberant naevus surrounded by a white halo (Figure 15). Over some months the naevus gradually disappears but the white patch stays for years. Often there are several such lesions and not infrequently the condition occurs alongside vitiligo.

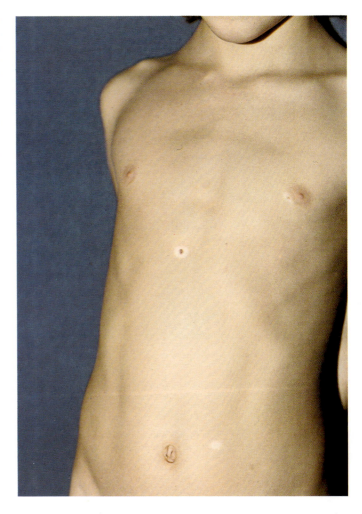

Figure 15 Sutton's naevus at different stages of evolution in a ten year old child. The lesion at the centre of the front of the chest shows a small papular naevus surrounded by a halo. The naevus on the left nipple has almost completely regressed, while in the umbilical region only a white (vitiliginous) spot remains, the naevus having disappeared.

Spitz naevus (juvenile melanoma)

This is an uncommon benign type of cellular naevus found in children and adolescents. Although there are some histological similarities to malignant melanoma, their biological relationship is unclear and some clinicians prefer not to use the term juvenile melanoma as it may cause anxiety and confusion. Characteristically these lesions are solitary red or red-brown in colour and often occur on the face. They have an initial period of rapid growth which then seems to decrease. However, their natural history is not well characterized as the diagnosis can only be established after they have been surgically removed. They may be mistaken for pyogenic granuloma (Figure 17). This last lesion often erodes and bleeds and it is only when this does not happen that confusion is likely to arise. Pressure will give rise to a dark colour in the case of a Spitz naevus but not a non-eroded pyogenic granuloma. Solitary xanthogranuloma may also be mistaken for a Spitz naevus, although the former usually has a yellowish colour (Figure 225).

Figure 16 Spitz naevus of the upper cheek in a one year old child.

Figure 17 Pyogenic granuloma. It has been sutured to stop the bleeding.

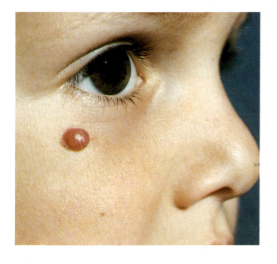

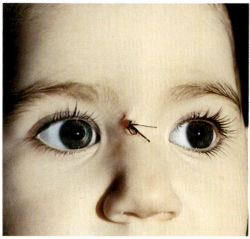

Epidermal naevus

This condition is the result of localized epidermal hypertrophy. It is apparent either at birth or within the first months of life. Clinically it presents as a localized, elongated, raised warty lesion (Figure 18). Occasionally, however, the condition may be systematized, occurring over most of the body (Figure 19). Apart from any aesthetic considerations, the condition may be associated with other congenital malformations – cardiac, bony, and so on. The main differential diagnosis is melanocytic naevus which can usually (but not always) be distinguished easily from epidermal naevus by its rounded, brown or black appearance and non-warty surface.

Treatment If the diagnosis is certain (biopsy may be necessary), localized lesions may be removed by surgical excision. The projecting part of larger lesions may be treated either by shaving the lesion parallel to the surface or by curettage. It should be noted that partial recurrences of the lesions may occur after any form of surgical treatment. Cryotherapy can also be useful at times.

Figure 18 Warty epidermal naevus of the scalp in a neonate.

Figure 19 Systematized warty epidermal naevus.

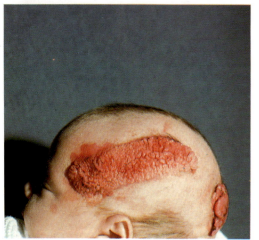

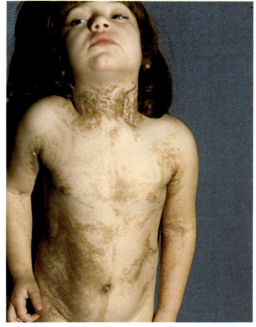

Naevus sebaceous

This is a localized hypertrophy of the sebaceous glands and other epidermal structures. Mostly it is present at birth and is localized on the scalp or face. Usually it presents as a yellowish-orange nodule, but it can be flat or just raised above the skin surface. On the scalp (Figure 20) it is usually hairless. At puberty the sebaceous tissue of the naevus shares in the generalized hypertrophy of sebaceous glands seen at this time and the lesions consequently become more prominent. When the lesion is a macule or barely raised above the skin surface the differential diagnosis can present difficulties. In particular it can be confused with alopecia areata or aplasia cutis, but the yellow colour and thickening of the skin should lead to the correct diagnosis.

The importance of naevus sebaceous is that the lesion gives rise to a malignant neoplasm of epithelial or glandular origin in up to 15 per cent of cases after the age of thirty. For this reason their removal before the third decade is often advised.

Figure 20 Sebaceous naevus of the scalp. The lesion is yellowish, hairless and just raised above the skin surface.

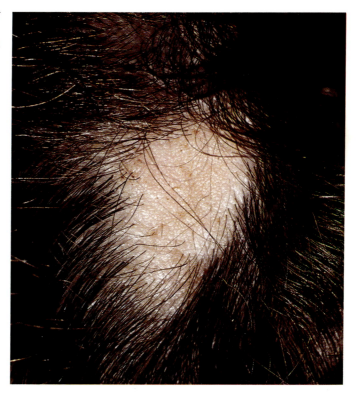

17

Haemangioma

This group of lesions is also naevoid and may be considered as benign neoplastic malformations. The lesions can originate from any component of primitive vascular tissue – arterial, venous, capillary or glomus tissue. Histologically the tissue of origin can usually be identified. However, it is not always possible or indeed desirable to biopsy these lesions, so that a clinical classification is also required. Clinically, smooth, raised and complex haemangiomas can be distinguished. Complex haemangiomas may be either smooth or raised but are accompanied by changes in deeper tissues or organs.

Raised haemangiomas

If one excludes common flat haemangiomas (salmon patches), the raised type are the most frequently occurring. When fully developed at between the ages of three and five months, they almost always have a superficial dermal component, and are know colloquially as strawberry naevi because of their fiery red colour. They may also have a deeper dermal and subcutaneous component evident as a skin-coloured swelling at the periphery of the lesion. This deeper component may have a bluish colour when the skin is stretched. There may be telangiectasia at the periphery of the lesion.

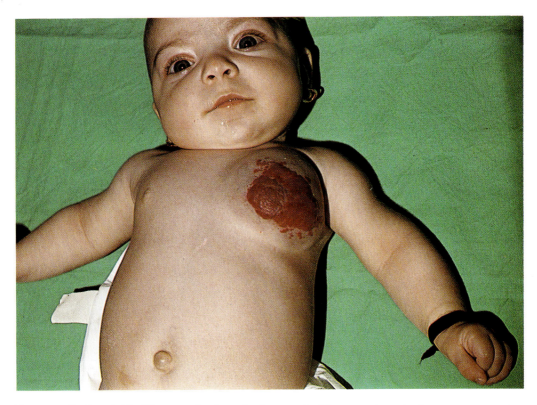

Figure 21 In this child of five months there is a large, raised haemangioma in the mammary region with a superficial intense red portion and a deeper, skin-coloured, subcutaneous component at the periphery.

Sites involved   Raised haemangiomas may occur anywhere but are most often found on the face and elsewhere in the head and neck region, and the upper limbs are more frequently involved than the lower. The site involved has prognostic importance.

Number of lesions   In more than 60 per cent the haemangioma is solitary. When there are many haemangiomas other organs may be involved, and the syndrome of disseminated intravascular coagulation may occur.

Natural history   They are present at birth in some 40 per cent of cases and most are evident by the second or third week of life. Rarely does a haemangioma appear later. When it does it tends not to regress spontaneously. Typically they start off as reddened, telangiectatic, flattened areas that remain static for the first month or so. Later, in the second month, the area tends to become raised and to develop its deeper component.

Haemangiomas of this type can grow at an alarming rate and this not unnaturally gives rise to parental anxiety. Sometimes these lesions grow to 10–20 cm in diameter. Generally the increase in size stops towards the end of the fourth month and they remain unchanged for the next few months.

When the infant reaches one year, further changes slowly begin. The bright red colour becomes paler, eventually to assume a whitish-grey appearance. This change usually begins at the centre and progresses centrifugally so that all that may remain is a peripheral red halo. As these changes in colour progress the whole lesion slowly decreases in size. This slow process of involution is usually complete in the first decade.

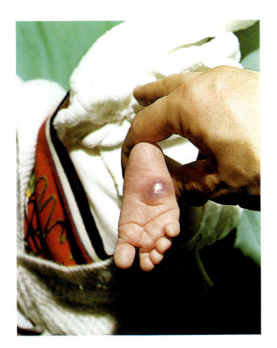

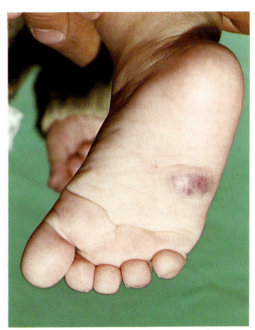

Figures 22, 23, 24 Raised haemangioma of the sole in a child of three months (Figure 22), at six months (Figure 23) and again at nine months (Figure 24). The apparently diminished intensity of the red colour of the lesion is due to the overlying thick plantar skin. The parents were worried that the lesion would interfere with walking, but their fears were groundless as the lesion regressed within the first year.

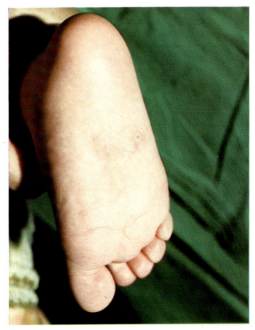

Smaller haemangiomas (2–3 cm in diameter) tend to regress completely and more rapidly, giving a cosmetically satisfactory end result. The larger lesions take longer to disappear but the eventual result is often surprisingly acceptable aesthetically. In some large lesions, lax dystrophic skin remains at the site after involution, but this is easily dealt with surgically.

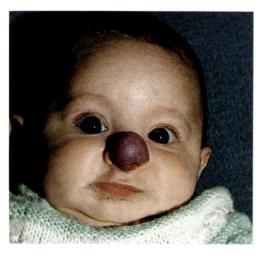

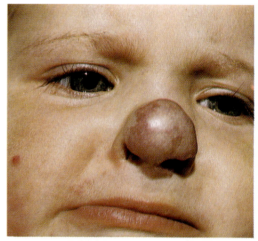

Figure 25 Raised haemangioma on the tip of the nose.

Figure 26 The same child as in Figure 25 now at the age of one year.

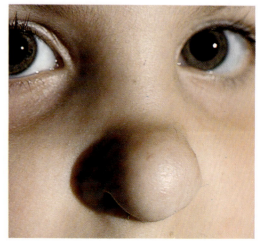

Figure 27 The same child as in Figures 25 and 26, now at four years of age. The angioma has spontaneously regressed.

Figure 28 Raised haemangioma of the cheek in a child of four months.

Figure 29 The same child at the age of one year.

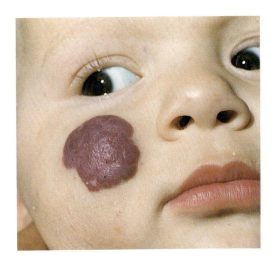

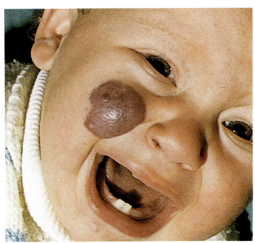

Figure 30 The same child at two years.

Figure 31 The same child at three years.

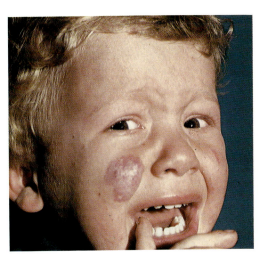

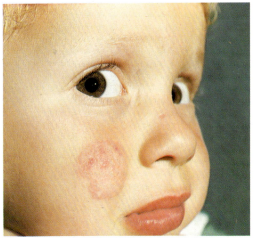

Complications

1. Ulceration and haemorrhage: the second of these is usually the result of the first. Ulceration occurs in about 5 per cent of lesions and is dependant on the site involved. Haemangiomas of the napkin region are particularly prone to this complication (Figure 32), presumably due to the chemical and mechanical trauma experienced in this region. Should haemorrhage occur, the result is not usually significant as it slows to a modest ooze within a few minutes. Ulceration is paradoxically a favourable sign, as the process of involution is accelerated as a result. However, residual scarring can result.

2. Compression of vital structures: this is a rare occurrence and occurs most frequently around the eye. At this site the eye itself may be

Figure 32 Ulcerated angioma of the buttock.

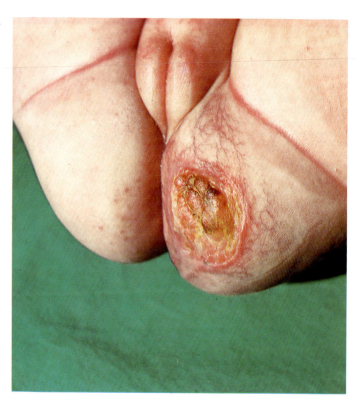

threatened or it may prevent adequate eye opening, causing visual disturbances, if that site is affected (Figure 33).

3. Failure of spontaneous regression: some 90 per cent of haemangiomas undergo spontaneous involution but in some case the lesion progresses to form large vascular lakes. This should be suspected if no regression is evident by the age of two. The lip (particularly the lower lip) is most often affected by this complication.

4. Disseminated intravascular coagulation (DIC): this complication is seen with very large haemangiomas or when there are multiple lesions. Subclinical DIC may occur and be evident only from laboratory studies.

Treatment Luckily the majority of raised haemangiomas regress spontaneously. For this reason it is unwise to initiate potentially hazardous or deforming treatments. Radiotherapy can interfere with local

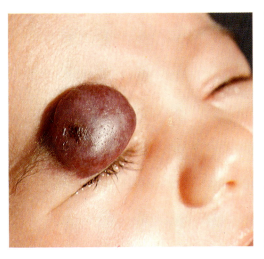

Figure 33 A palpebral angioma can cause visual disturbances.

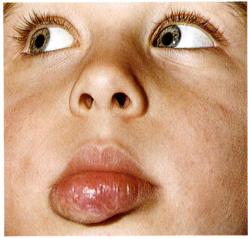

Figure 34 Haemangioma of the lower lip that has failed to regress.

bone growth and may even be responsible for sarcomatous change in the angioma. Because of the tendency to spontaneous regression, surgery is only needed to correct any residual malformation or improve the cosmetic defect that remains.

Cryotherapy may help to promote involution in an angioma, especially if it is on an exposed site. This type of treatment must be superficial and of short duration (three to four seconds only with a standard cryoprobe) to avoid unnecessary pain and discomfort and subsequent ulceration.

Treatment with sclerosants is dangerous and should be avoided. It should be reserved as an alternative to surgical intervention in those few patients whose angioma does not regress spontaneously and in which, presumably, there are widely dilated vascular channels.

Treatment with systemic steroids can be used for patients whose angiomas are growing rapidly in awkward anatomical areas (Figure 35), for example, those around the eyes. Prednisone is given in a dose of 2–4 mg/kg per day for the entire period of growth of the angioma – usually two to three months, then gradually withdrawn. To avoid the unpleasant side effects of steroid therapy this form of treatment is reserved for patients with gross lesions producing a functional defect. It must be emphasized that in the majority of patients the best treatment is no treatment.

There is an obvious need to reassure the parents, who are often given confusing and conflicting advice by all and sundry. It is often helpful to show them pictures of patients before and after the spontaneous

Figure 35 Patient with deep angioma involving the nasal bones, for which systemic steroids were indicated.

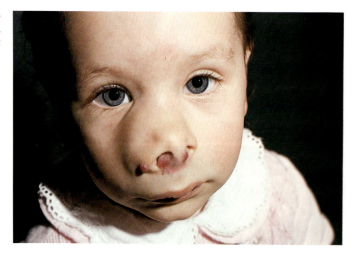

resolution of lesions – and this is particularly useful if the pictures relate to haemangiomas in the same site as in their own child. In the first six months it is worthwhile seeing the child monthly to measure and photograph the lesion. The measurements and photographs can then be shown to the parents on successive visits to demonstrate the reduction of size.

It is useful to keep larger, protuberant lesions covered with an elasticated bandage in order to avoid the lesion expanding and to prevent mechanical problems.

Smooth haemangiomas

In 50 per cent of newborn babies there are angiomas at birth (salmon patches). The site most frequently involved is the nape of the neck, but the central part of the forehead and the eyebrow region are also affected. Most rarely other sites may be affected. The lesions on the face tend to resolve, but those on the nape of the neck, which are anyway more prominent, persist through life and become obvious when there is hair loss.

Spider naevi are composed of a central vascular channel, and are characterized by a central smooth-surfaced protuberance, from which

Figure 36 Spider naevus on back of hand.

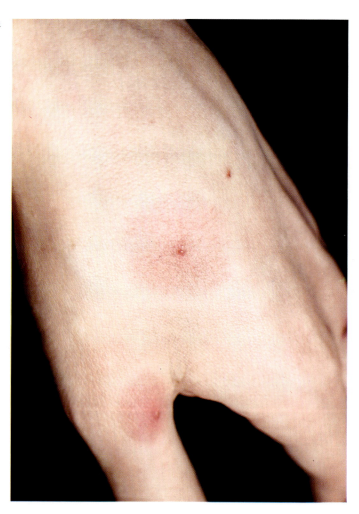

radiates telangiectatic blood vessels. They tend to occur in light exposed sites and only in skin whose venous drainage is into the superior vena cava. Although they are frequently found in normal, healthy individuals they also occur in alcoholic cirrhosis and during pregnancy. Electrocoagulation of the central vascular channel is usually sufficient for their removal.

Smooth haemangiomas tend to persist unchanged for life and are resistant to treatment. The most notable example is the naevus flammeus or port wine stain which usually has the distribution of a dorsal nerve root (Figure 37). After some years the initial crimson-red colour becomes darker and more cyanotic and the surface may become rugose due to the formation of angiomatous nodules (Figure 37). Treatment for these lesions has been unsatisfactory, as mentioned previously, but recent reports of the successful use of the argon laser offers new hope for at least some affected individuals. Laser treatment is most useful after the age of twenty, as the coagulative action of the laser helps most when there are larger vascular channels present.

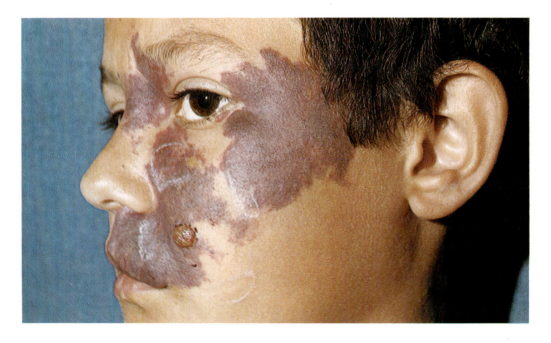

Figure 37 Port wine stain with angiomatous nodule in trigeminal distribution. Note that the upper eyelid is little involved and there was no intracranial angiomatous component in this patient.

Complex haemangiomas

Haemangiomatous hypertrophy of skin overlying a limb may be associated with the hypertrophy of the underlying bony structure due to the increased rate of blood flow through the affected area. The condition varies in severity from those in which it is incompatible with life (Figure 38) to less severe cases in which asymmetry of the limb is just evident (Figures 39, 40) and is non-progressive and compatible with a normal life.

In the Sturge-Weber syndrome (cerebro-cutaneous angiomatosis) a

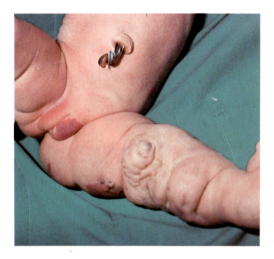

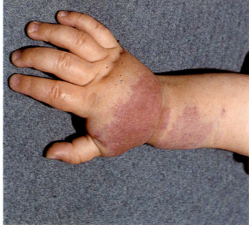

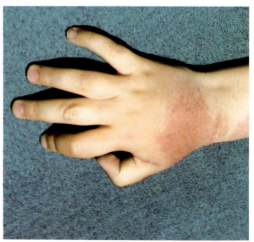

Figure 38 Grave haemangiomatous hypertrophy in a neonate with obviously dilated superficial vessels and considerable arteriovenous shunting.

Figure 39 Mild haemangiomatous hypertrophy at the age of six months.

Figure 40 The same child as in Figure 39 at four years of age.

port wine stain of the face is associated with an angiomatous malformation of the underlying meninges. This association is particularly frequent when the upper eyelid is completely covered by the angioma (Figure 41).

Angiomas of other organs should be suspected in the presence of multiple cutaneous angiomata (Figure 42). Life-threatening hepatic angioma may present clinically as cardiac failure and should then be treated by systemic corticosteroids.

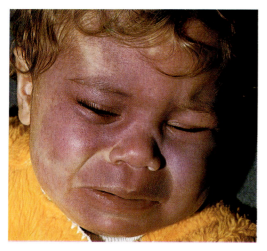

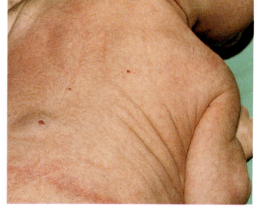

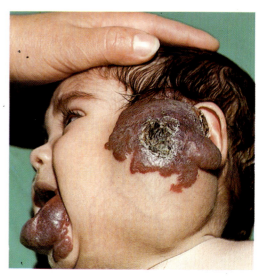

Figure 41 Sturge-Weber syndrome. The port wine stain affects the whole face, including the forehead.

Figure 42 Multiple angiomata associated with the disseminated intravascular coagulation syndrome.

Figure 43 Severe cutaneo-laryngeal angiomatosis. Note the involvement of the lower lip.

Systemic corticosteriods should also be used for cutaneo-laryngeal angiomatosis (Figure 43). This condition should be suspected in the presence of angiomata of the lip and buccal cavity when there is stridor and/or dyspnoea (Figure 44).

Figure 44 Cutaneo-laryngeal angiomatosis. Inspirational dyspnoea has produced collapse of the thoracic cage.

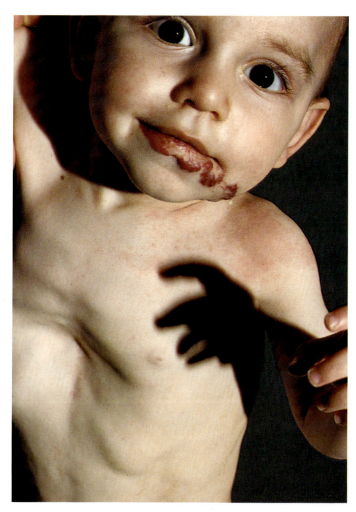

Superficial pyoderma

This type of infection of the skin is caused by pyogenic cocci – most frequently staphylococcus aureus. Various clinical pictures may result, including folliculitis, impetigo contagiosa and bullous impetigo and impetiginization of other dermatoses.

Impetigo contagiosa and bullous impetigo are the most frequent bacterial infection of the skin in infancy. They typically occur before the age of ten. Bullae containing a serous fluid often form on the affected area. Lesions may occur in the inguinal and perianal regions in very young infants (Figure 45). In older children lesions are more frequently found around the mouth, nose and eyes (Figure 46).

The first sign of the disorder is often the appearance of small vesicles (1 to 2 mm diameter) which rupture to form moist erosions which rapidly extend at the periphery. The rapid peripheral extension of vesicles and bullae is quite characteristic, distinguishing the disorder from other bullous complaints of childhood. The lesions usually extend asymmetrically and the bullae, which often coalesce, eventually dry to give rise to a golden-yellowish or greenish-yellow crust (Figure 46). After a few days the crusts separate, leaving a discoloured area of skin.

Figure 45 Bullous pyoderma in a two month old child. Note that there is a bulla in the pubic region and extensive moist erosions with scalloped borders.

Figure 46 Child of four with a bullous pyoderma of the face. The initial lesion is larger and in the perioral area. The subsequent lesions are smaller.

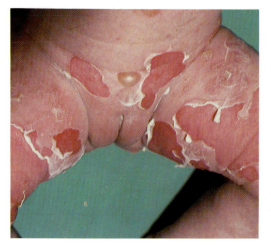

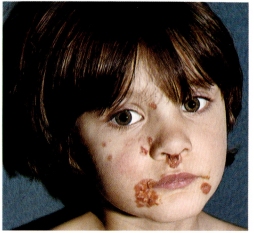

The disease is caused by pyogenic cocci – most frequently staphylococcus aureus. It is very contagious and spreads rapidly in hot, humid climates. Most cases consist of a few localized lesions which rapidly respond to topical treatment. A few children (especially in the neonatal period) are much more seriously affected by a widespread or generalized disorder. This condition is know as toxic epidermal necrolysis (or the staphylococcal scalded skin syndrome) and is characterized by sheeted desquamation and thin, flaccid blisters (Figure 47). The typical peeling seen is the result of sloughing of the most superficial part of the epidermis and is due to an exotoxin produced by certain groups of staphylococci – particularly Group II phage type 71.

A similar syndrome clinically is occasionally seen in older children and adults and may be due to drug hypersensitivity. It is important to distinguish this disorder from the staphylococcal scalded skin syndrome as

Figure 47 One year old child with toxic epidermal necrolysis. Note the extensive superficial exfoliation.

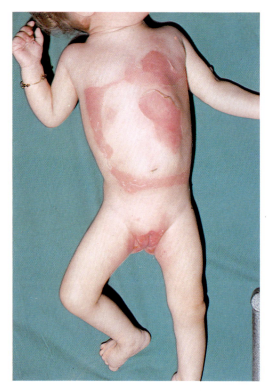

antibiotics are required for the latter disease and corticosteroids for the drug-induced disorder.

Treatment   Localized bullous impetigo should always be treated with topical antimicrobials and antiseptic cleansers such as hypochlorite solution or povidone-iodine preparations. Ointments containing antibiotics are also sometimes prescribed. However, it is probably best to administer antibiotics systemically (penicillin or erythromycin preferably) to all patients save those with only one or two small localized areas.

Pyogenic bacteria can also cause other disorders such as folliculitis and boils, as well as secondary impetiginization of other dermatoses including atopic eczema, dyshidrotic eczema of the feet, pediculosis capitis, scabies and papular uriticaria. Sweat gland abscesses of the scalp may occur in infancy (Figure 48).

Figure 48 Suppurative miliaria of the scalp in an infant.

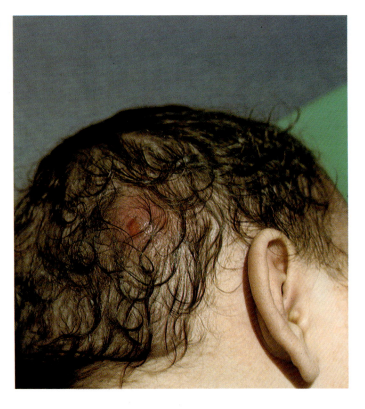

Erysipelas is rare in young children (Figure 49) as is bacterial paronychia (Figure 50). These disorders usually present in later childhood, although monilial paronychia is sometimes seen. Paronychia usually responds to similar local treatment as impetigo (see above) but systemic antibiotics are often indicated when the condition is acute or several fingers are involved.

Figure 49 Erysipelas secondary to eczema of the foot.

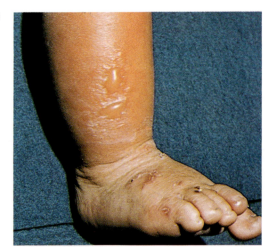

Figure 50 Bacterial paronychia with secondary nail deformity in a child of nine months.

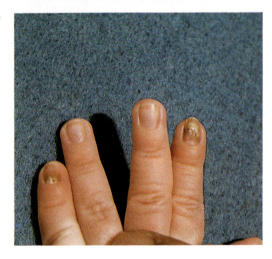

Congenital syphilis

Syphilis is one of the disorders, alongside leprosy and tuberculosis, that prior to effective treatment caused great fear and prejudice. Interestingly, the prejudice lingers on as part of the general primitive fear of contagion engendered by all skin diseases. When diagnosed early on, syphilis is easily cured by penicillin, to which, miraculously, it is still sensitive. Early diagnosis is important but can be difficult.

If the disease is missed, irreversible damage may occur and give rise to the serious classical 'tertiary' manifestations of the disorder in later years. Failure to detect syphilis in women can also result in congenital syphilis from the intranatal infection of an infant. A recent American study has determined that one neonate in 2,500 is affected by congenital syphilis unknown to either parents or doctor – an incidence similar to that of congenital hypothyroidism. In Italy, the frequency of unknown congenital syphilis is probably greater than the observed levels in the USA as has been demonstrated by a similar study. In the UK the frequency is 0.35 per 100,000 live births.

For these reasons it is vital to ensure that the general public are aware of the problem and that they and the administration recognize the importance of screening tests for syphilis in pregnancy. Similarly, education of the young about venereal disorders and their prevention should also reduce the risk. An infected mother is infectious only in the early stages of the disease and can pass it to the foetus only after the fourth month of pregnancy when the placenta is well formed. The effect on the foetus depends on the severity of the infection and the age at which infection occurs. Spontaneous abortion or premature delivery can occur, as can stillbirth. It can also present in the first few months of life with symptoms referable to any organ.

More frequently presentations include haemolytic anaemia, hepatosplenomegaly, persistent rhinitis and various types of skin lesion. Palmar-plantar lesions are often seen and may be bullous (syphilitic pemphigus) or papular (Figure 51). Syphilitic papules may also occur in other sites in other regions such as the perianal region (Figure 52) where they may be differentiated from condyloma acuminatum from viral infection. Papules may also be seen over the limbs (Figures 53, 54). Syphilis infection can also result in an osteochondritis and cause a pseudoparalysis (Parrot's pseudoparalysis, Figure 53).

Figure 51 Plantar syphiloderma in a neonate. Papular lesions are present.

Figure 52 Syphilitic papules in the perianal region.

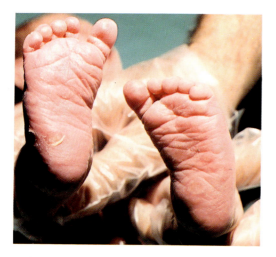

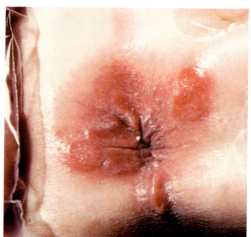

Figure 53 Pseudoparalysis of an arm due to syphilitic osteochondritis.

Figure 54 Detail to show papular syphiloderma.

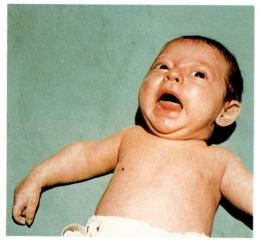

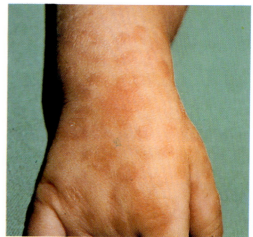

Diagnosis   Congenital syphilis diagnosis rests on its recognition clinically and confirmation by the appropriate laboratory tests. A particular difficulty in the laboratory diagnosis of syphilis in the neonate lies in the differentiation of a positive test such as the VDRL due to the passive transplacental transmission of maternal antibodies caused by previous (and cured) infection of the mother and true congenital syphilis. When the positive test is due to a previous, cured infection the neonate is healthy and the antibodies disappear from the circulation in a few months. Some tests (such as the FTA/1gM195) can differentiate the two situations.

Treatment   For congenital syphilis this is still based on the use of penicillin as it is still the most effective and least toxic agent for this much feared disorder. If the central nervous system is not affected, slow-acting penicillin can be used (benzathine penicillin) in a dose of 50,000 iu/kg in eight to ten intramuscular injections over a month. Some believe that a single dose of benzathine penicillin is sufficient. If, however, the CSF shows evidence of infection, soluble penicillin should be used in a dose of 50,000 iu/kg per day in divided doses for ten to fifteen days. If for any reason adequate examination of the CSF is not possible a mixture of benzathine and soluble penicillin should be given.

Coxsackie virus infections

Herpangina occurs in school aged children as a short-lived, febrile illness which does not recur. The onset is sudden, with high fever for four or five days and is accompanied by small vesicles (1 to 2 mm in diameter) in the mouth and pharynx. The condition is painful and makes eating difficult. The condition has to be distinguished from hand, foot and mouth disease (Figure 55), but in herpangina there are no skin lesions and more systemic disturbance. It must also be distinguished from herpetic stomatitis, in which there may be severe systemic upset and marked oral discomfort. In the latter the lesions are more often localized to the front of the mouth with lesions on the skin of and around the lips. It is easier to differentiate the other disorders of this region (see Table 1).

Table 1
Differential diagnosis of disorders of the oral cavity

	Herpangina	Hand, foot and mouth	Primary herpetic stomatitis	Apthosis	Fixed drug eurption
Fever	40%	38%	40%	No	No
Infectivity	Yes	Sometimes	No	No	No
Involvement of back of mouth	Yes	Yes	No	Yes	Yes
Skin lesions	No	Yes	Yes	No	Often
Recurrences	No	No	No	Yes	Yes
Difficulty in swallowing	Severe	Mild	Severe	Mild	Severe

Hand, foot and mouth disease varies in incidence in different countries and in different regions of the same country. It is caused by Coxsackie A16 or more rarely by other viruses of the same group. It occurs either in minor epidemics or sporadically. It is characterized by the appearance of elongated pustules on the hands, feet and knees and more rarely of other sites. Similar lesions to those of herpangina involve the oral cavity (Figure 55) and the skin around the mouth. There is little systemic upset.

Figure 55 Hand, foot and mouth disease. Oral and perioral vesicles.

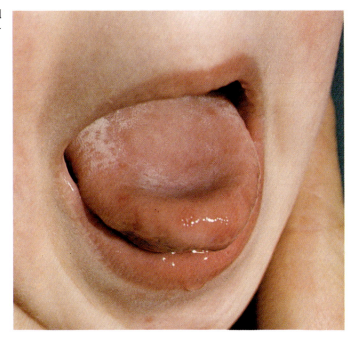

Figure 56 Hand, foot and mouth disease. Characteristic elongated pustules of the hand and of the knee.

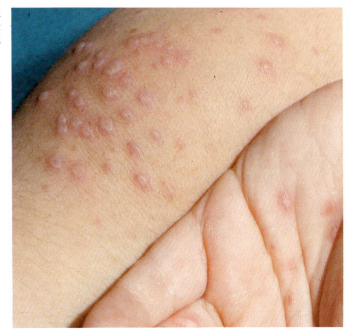

Verrucae and condylomata acuminata

Verrucae (or common viral warts) are benign epidermal neoplasms caused by a papova virus infection. Viruses of the same group but which possess minor antigenic differences cause morphologically different lesions. Plane warts, filiform warts, plantar warts, ordinary verrucae vulgares and condylomata acuminata are examples of lesions caused by different antigenic types of wart viruses.

Plane warts (Figure 57) are more frequent in early childhood but by no means confined to this age group. They are frequently found on the face

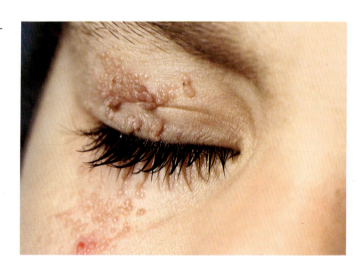

Figure 57 Warts of upper eyelid.

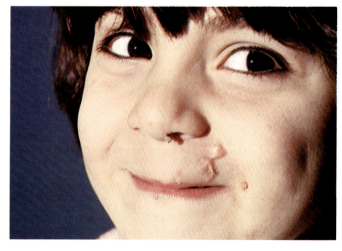

Figure 58 Filiform warts of nose and scar from diathermy.

and may be present in large numbers, making treatment difficult. Rarely, these lesions may be confused with those of benign histiocytic disorder but lesions in the latter are usually yellowish in colour (Figure 227).

Filiform warts (Figure 58) are usually found on the face around one of its orifices. Common warts or verrucae vulgares (Figures 59, 60) are raised and tend to have a cauliflower-like surface. Mostly they occur on the hands. Plantar warts are usually tender to pressure and may be differentiated from corns by the presence of closely set black dots on their surface representing the tips of dermal papillae. There may be a familial predisposition to multiple warts which recur. In some patients of this sort (Figure 60) an immune deficiency can be demonstrated.

Genital warts (condylomata acuminata) are caused by a member of the same group of papova viruses (Figures 61, 62, 63) and are characteristically localized to the genital mucosae or perianal skin. They are usually spread venereally and often occur in association with other venereal disorders. However, this is not true where children are concerned, in whom they are mostly seen perianally. Mothers of children with the disorder may have common warts of the hands but of course this may be a chance association (Figure 61). Individual susceptibility to the wart virus varies – the same

Figure 59 Common warts of the hands and penis.

Figure 60 Numerous recurrent common warts in a child with atopic dermatitis who had a deficiency of cellular immunity.

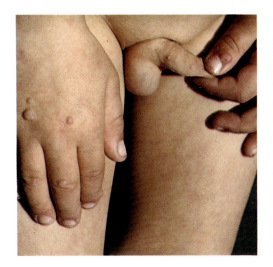

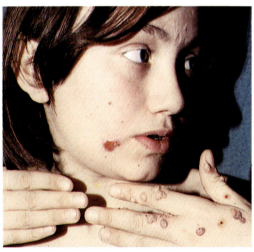

virus causing differing problems in different hosts (Figure 62).

Evolution   All forms of warts tend to persist for long periods and to recur after treatment – especially in those with numerous lesions who seem to cope inadequately with virus infections. Warts can also regress spontaneously (Figures 64, 65).

Figure 61 Common warts of hand in mother and perianal condylomata acuminata in her son.

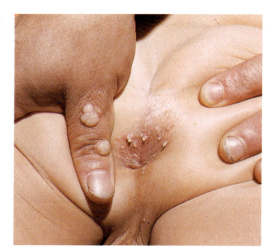

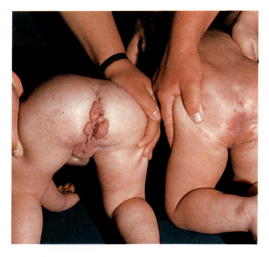

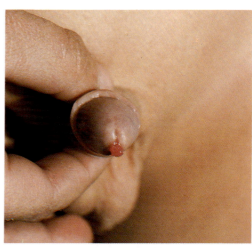

Figure 62 Perianal condyloma acuminata of different types in identical twins.

Figure 63 Condyloma acuminata of urethral orifice in a child of four years.

Treatment There is no specific antiviral compound for the treatment of warts. Management is largely a matter of deciding if and when the warts should be removed by one or another destructive treatment. As whatever is done there is a high risk of recurrence, it is important not to cause pain in the child. Removal by curette after producing local anaesthesia may be suitable for isolated warts or when there are only a few present. Liquid nitrogen, solid carbon dioxide (or a cryoprobe instrument) may also be used.

It is important not to attempt extensive invasive procedures for removal requiring multiple local injections for anaesthesia or a general anaesthetic. It must be remembered that warts are benign, they remit spontaneously, and all forms of treatment are bedevilled by recurrences. In addition, surgical removal can lead to postoperative infection and scarring. Facial plane warts and condylomata acuminata are often very numerous. They may be treated with preparations of podophyllin in tinctures of flexible collodior film (5–25 per cent). Preparations containing 5-Fluorouacil (5 per cent in cream) may also be employed. Caution is required with both of these local applications as the active ingredients may be absorbed and cause serious systemic toxicity (podophyllin has caused fatalities). These treatments can also cause considerable local irritation of the surrounding

Figure 64 Common warts of the left hand and the chest wall.

Figure 65 Spontaneous regression of warts seen in Figure 64.

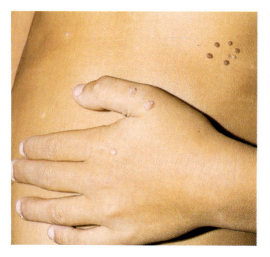

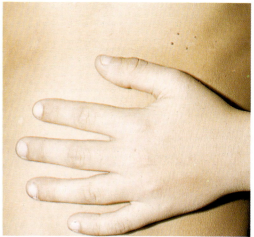

skin. Topical salicylic acid-containing preparations (16–33 per cent) may be applied once daily for two to four weeks.

Some lesions remit spontaneously after several years of being stubbornly resistant to all treatment.

Viruses of the herpes group: varicella

Most important illnesses due to viruses of this group are caused either by herpes simplex virus (HSV) or by the varicella zoster virus (VZV). These two very different viruses infect nearly everyone and cause two groups of disorders whose clinical signs differ quite markedly. Both viruses may cause a generalized disorder in a subject who has not been previously infected and has no immune defence to the infecting agent (for example, chicken pox – varicella). However, primary infection with HSV may not be clinically evident and when it is it may cause a variety of clinical states, including a severe widespread vesicular rash, herpetic gingivostomatitis and generalized herpes infection superimposed on atopic dermatitis. Both viruses persist in the tissues for long periods and can cause secondary manifestations later. The VZV causes herpes zoster in immune individuals and HSV causes repeated episodes of a herpetiform rash. Herpes zoster is not generally recurrent.

The VZV causes varicella (chicken pox) in non-immune individuals. Varicella is easy to recognize in the typical case in an epidemic but may be

Figure 66 Lesions of chicken pox.

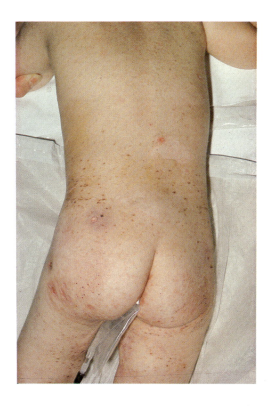

more difficult in the older child or adult when occurring sporadically. The primary lesion is usually a pustule some 2 mm in diameter and surrounded by erythema. The lesions may be quite inflamed with considerable redness and swelling (Figure 66). The lesions of chicken pox may be confused with insect bites or even banal folliculitis (Figure 67).

Treatment   Usually chicken pox is a quite benign disorder not requiring special treatment. However, in patients who are immunologically compromised (such as those with leukaemia), a severe and even fatal haemorrhagic form can occur (Figure 68). The disease is only contagious in the first few days, but it is advisable to keep the young patient at home until all the crusts have separated (three or four weeks). Usually symptomatic treatment with bland or antiseptic lotions is sufficient. Gammaglobulin may be indicated for those with an immuno-deficiency.

Figure 67 Lesions of chicken pox without surrounding erythema.

Figure 68 Severe haemorrhagic chicken pox in a leukaemic infant girl.

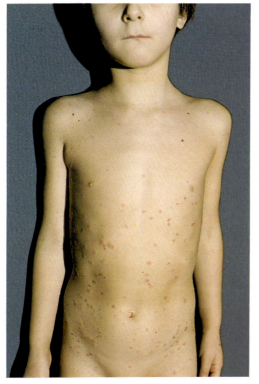
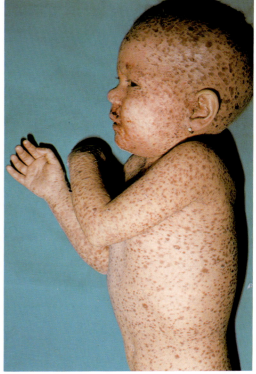

Herpes zoster

Herpes zoster (shingles) is due to infection of a localized area of skin with the varicella zoster virus in someone who has previously had chicken pox and has circulating antibodies. Herpes zoster is rare in the first ten years of life and when it does occur at this time is not a severe illness. Immunocompromised children seem more prone to contract the disorder and in this group it may be quite severe. As in the adult, herpes zoster occurs unilaterally in the distribution of a dorsal nerve root (Figures 69, 70, 71). Herpes zoster in paediatric patients is distinguished by the complete absence of pain. In older children the degree of pain experienced is proportional to the age.

The disorder may be extremely serious in children with neoplastic disease or who are for some reason immunosuppressed, and may become

Figure 69 Herpes zoster of the thigh of a child aged three. Note that the child is smiling and not in obvious pain.

Figure 70 Recurrent shingles in a leukaemic child aged eight. Note that the right scapula region is hypopigmented from a previous attack.

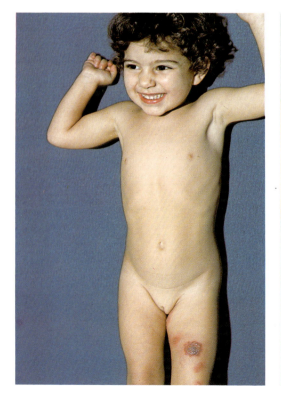

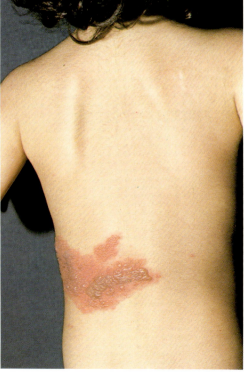

haemorrhagic or necrotic (Figure 71) in this group. Typical vesiculo-pustules of chicken pox (herpes zoster varicellosus) may appear in large numbers elsewhere in children who have a defect in their immune defences, demonstrating the importance of the immune system in the usually local nature of herpes zoster. The diagnosis or herpes zoster does not usually cause any difficulty, although it has to be distinguished in a few cases from generalized herpes simplex.

In an otherwise normal child with localized herpes zoster, local treatment with an antiseptic such as povidone-iodine is all that is required. However, when the disease occurs in an immunocompromised subject who is severely ill, intravenous acyclovir may be given as it has been reported that this shortens the complaint and appears to diminish its severity.

Figure 71 Gangrenous herpes zoster in a leukaemic child.

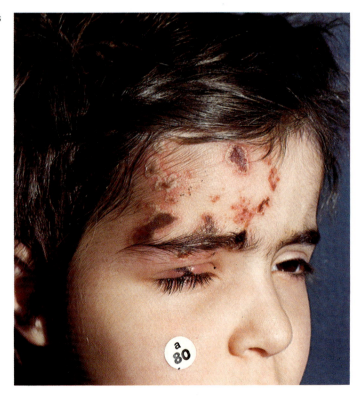

Herpes simplex

When primary infection with herpes simplex is evident clinically it may give rise to a serious systemic disorder. The most frequent dermatological presentations of primary herpes simplex infection are gingivostomatitis or a herpetic superinfection in children with eczema. Gingivostomatitis (Figure 72) is characterized by necrotic and pustular lesions of the anterior part of the oral cavity, of the tongue and of the lips and adjoining skin. The disorder is accompanied by fever, malaise and difficulty in eating and drinking. For differential diagnosis, see page 40. Herpetic superinfection (Figures 73, 74, 75, 76) occurs in children with pre-existing eczematous disorders – usually atopic dermatitis, who have been in contact with someone with recurrent herpes simplex.

Figure 72 Herpetic gingivostomatitis with perioral and facial pustular lesions.

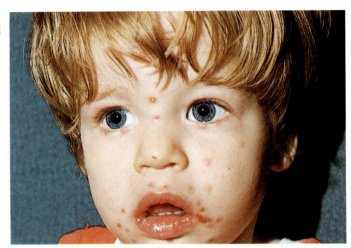

Figure 73 Herpetic superinfection of atopic dermatitis with typical clusters of herpetic lesions.

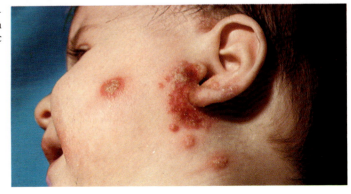

Figure 74 Labial herpes simplex in mother and simultaneous herpetic superinfection of her son's cheeks affected by atopic dermatitis.

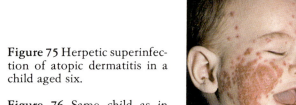

Figure 75 Herpetic superinfection of atopic dermatitis in a child aged six.

Figure 76 Same child as in Figure 75 eighteen days later with atopic dermatitis of the face and antecubital fossae.

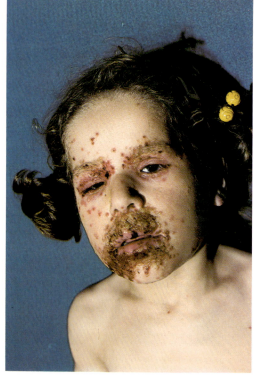

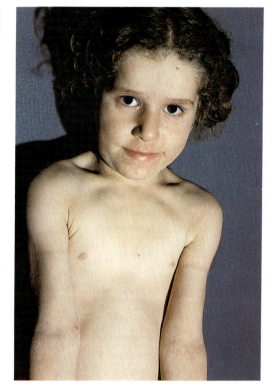

Primary herpes simplex can be an extremely serious disorder which can give rise to complications in the central nervous system and may even be fatal.

After primary infection the virus remains dormant in the sensory ganglia but retraces its steps along the sensory nerves to the skin after a traumatic stimulus of some kind. The presence of circulating antibodies ensures that the disorder remains localized in post-primary recurrent attacks. In the child the area most frequently involved by recurrent herpes simplex infection is the cheek (Figures 77, 78) while in the adult it is the

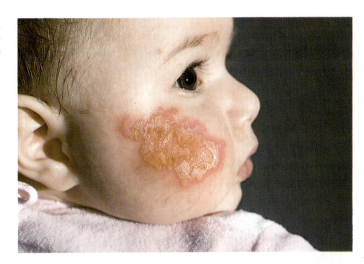

Figure 77 Clusters of typical pustules and papulovesicles due to recurrent herpes simplex.

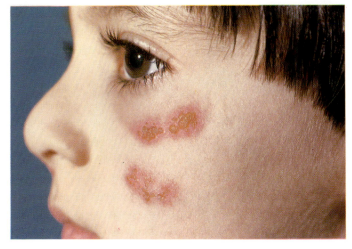

Figure 78 Herpes simplex of the cheek. Eroded lesions and papulovesicles and pustules in clusters.

perilabial area and the labial mucosa itself that are usually affected. Interestingly adults with recurrent herpes simplex rarely give a history of herpes simplex in infancy.

Typically, the recurrent disorder is unilateral and presents as well defined clusters of papulovesicles and pustules. Although the zygomatic area is the most frequently involved site, other parts of the skin may be affected (Figures 79, 80). After a few days erosions develop which later become crusted (Figure 78). Following separation of the crusts, discoloured areas remain which occasionally are atrophic or even more definitely scarred. The well-defined clustered arrangement of lesions is still easily visible at this stage. These clinical features are quite consistent and allow the diagnosis to be made easily.

Recurrences can happen as often as every fifteen to twenty days or as infrequently as once or twice per year. They are more frequent in the winter time in association with upper respiratory tract infections or other pyrexial episodes.

Figure 79 Thumb affected by recurrent herpes simplex.

Figure 80 Recurrent herpes simplex of the penis.

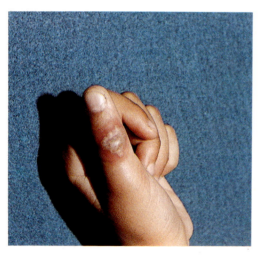

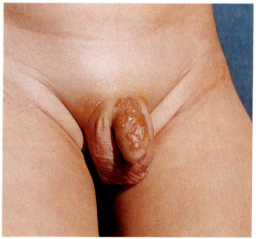

Recurrent herpes simplex in childhood is important from a number of standpoints. Firstly, it is one of the ten most common skin diseases seen in this age group. Secondly, it causes considerable discomfort and embarrassment over many years. If the disorder recurs repeatedly at the same site, permanent scarring may occur. Herpes simplex sometimes involves the palpebral region and then may affect the eye, causing a keratitis with subsequent corneal opacities (Figure 82). Ocular involvement occurs in approximately 8 per cent of patients with recurrent herpes simplex.

Figure 81 Recurring herpes simplex of palpebral region.

Figure 82 Corneal opacities due to herpetic keratitis.

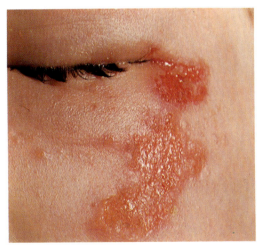

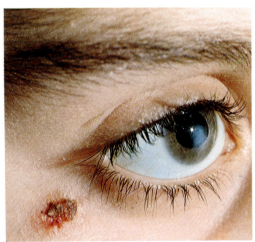

Treatment   Local treatment with antiseptics and 5-deoxyuridine does not stop recurrences. Treatment with preparations containing the drug acyclovir have been reported to shorten the duration of attacks and also decrease the period of 'viral shedding'. It has not been substantiated that they lessen the frequency of recurrences. Attempts to decrease the frequency of recurrences with immunostimulants, including levamisole, TP5 and transfer factor, or by repeated vaccination, have not been substantiated.

Molluscum contagiosum

This disorder is a further example of a virally induced nodule. It occurs mainly in the first decade, although other age groups are not immune. The primary lesion is a white, pink or red papule 1–3 mm in diameter (or occasionally larger) with a central umbilication containing a plug of greyish debris. Lesions often occur over the face in variable numbers and can be quite difficult to recognize. They disappear spontaneously as do warts, but appear to do so more readily than warts. They may occasionally become inflamed and subsequently regress. They may also develop an area of eczema around them, the significance of which is uncertain.

Treatment   There is no specific treatment but they can be dealt with by expression of the central plug of horny debris or by some form of local destructive therapy, for example, cautery.

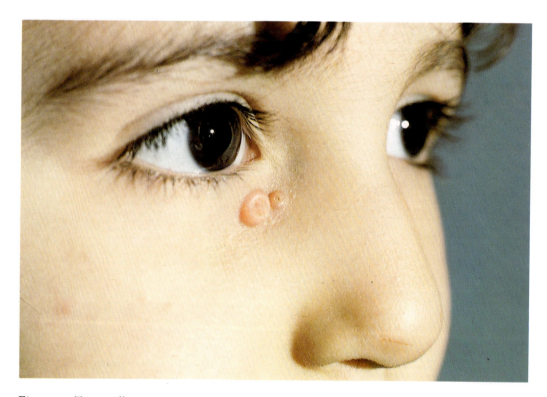

Figure 83 Two mullusca contagiosa on the face. Note the central umbilications.

Cat scratch fever

This is a fairly uncommon disorder due to a bedsonia type of micro-organism which is usually transmitted by a cat scratch. It mainly affects infants who play with cats and a history of a scratch from the pet is quite common.

After a ten-day incubation period a banal papule or nodule appears on the forearm (Figure 84) or back of the hand or thigh. A regional lymphadenopathy follows which is disproportionately severe when compared with the original lesion. When the initial lesion is not prominent it is difficult to recognize and the lymphadenopathy that

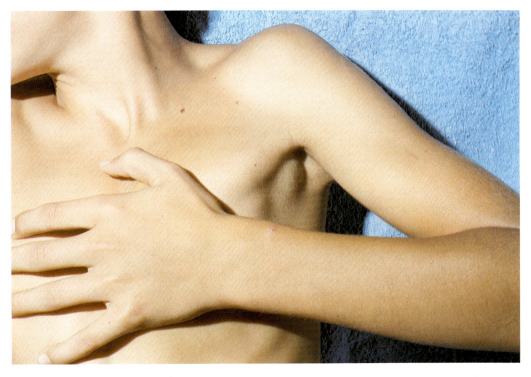

Figure 84 Cat scratch fever with prominent axillary lymphadenopathy. Note the banal nodular lesion on the radial border of the wrist.

ensues often causes diagnostic difficulty. In such cases the initial cutaneous lesion must be carefully looked for. The lymphadenopathy sometimes proceeds to suppuration although resolution usually occurs in two to six weeks, even when the glandular enlargement is very marked.

Pityriasis rosea

Many of the features of this disorder suggest a viral aetiology but this has never been substantiated. It mostly affects individuals in their teens and twenties, but is by no means restricted to them as it is occasionally seen in younger children and the elderly. It often occurs in small epidemics in the spring or autumn.

Characteristically the disorder starts with a large scaling pink macule on the trunk (herald patch) (Figure 85). A few days later numerous other smaller, similar lesions appear over the trunk and sometimes the proximal parts of the limbs. Generally the eruption is asymptomatic with little itchiness. The disease usually remits spontaneously after four to eight weeks.

The diagnosis depends on both the clinical morphology and history. Typically the periphery of each macular lesion is redder and more scaly that the central region. The macules tend to be oval and are often distributed in a 'Christmas tree' like arrangement along the ribs symmetrically.

Treatment This may not be necessary although if there is some discomfort a bland emollient may be prescribed.

Figure 85 Typical pityriasis rosea on the trunk.

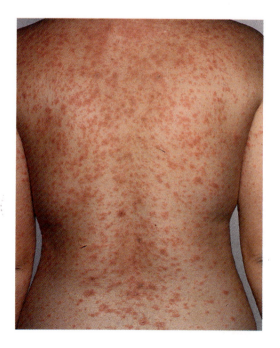

Guttate parapsoriasis (pityriasis lichenoides)

The aetiology of this disorder is unknown but some of its features suggest that it is the result of a cutaneous vasculitis secondary to a viral infection. It has some clinical similarities to chicken pox and has been termed varicelliform parapsoriasis (pityriasis lichenoides et varioliformis acuta). The lesions are polymorphic but generally are papular to start with and develop a central necrotic and exudative area. In some lesions this central change is minimal and results only in a characteristic scale which is attached centrally but free peripherally (mica scale) so that it can easily be removed. In other papules the necrosis causes a purple or black scab to appear (Figure 86). Lesions are variable in number and can occur anywhere but are more prolific on the trunk and limbs. The course of the complaint is characteristically relapsing and may last several years.

There is no systemic disturbance and no typical laboratory findings, although biopsy of the lesions may reveal quite characteristic histological findings. When a patient first presents, the disease has to be distinguished from chicken pox and from pityriasis rosea but, as indicated, these two disorders last for much shorter periods.

Treatment   Systemic and topical treatments have no effect on the course of the disorder. Patients often report that their rash improves at least temporarily in the sun and, if necessary, ultraviolet treatment can be administered in patients with an extensive eruption. PUVA (photo-chemotherapy with long wave ultraviolet light and prior administration of psoralen) has also been reported as helpful for some patients.

Figure 86 Guttate parapsoriasis. Note crusted lesions in the pectoral region.

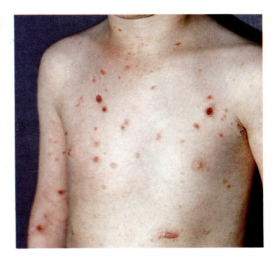

Viral eruptions

A frequent diagnostic problem is the presence of a widespread exanthematic rash which may be viral in origin or drug-induced. Leaving aside chicken pox and measles, which are generally not in doubt diagnostically, the other virally caused rashes are not dramatic. For example, roseola (Figure 87) presents with mild fever and cervical lymphadenopathy (which may be diagnostically useful) but a non-specific eruption which can make identification difficult. Confirmation of the diagnosis can only be made by the detection of a raised titre of antibodies some fifteen days after the illness. A quite typical 'roseola' like eruption can be provoked by ampicillin (Figure 88).

Figure 87 Roseola. Note lymph node enlargement at the sides of the neck.

Figure 88 Roseoliform eruption from ampicillin.

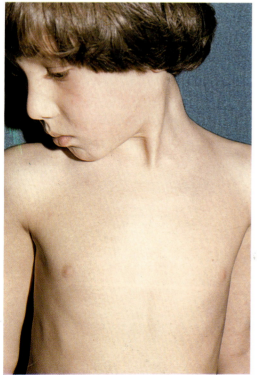

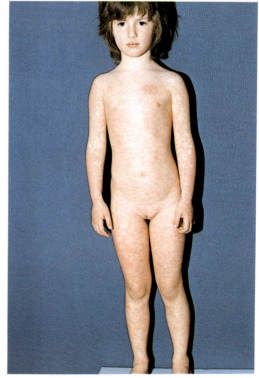

The presence of a similar eruption (or history of one in the previous two weeks) in family and friends (Figure 89) strongly suggests a viral aetiology, the absence of systemic symptoms favours provocation by a drug. Other features that will aid pinpointing a drug as the cause include a history of an identical eruption previously and the taking of an ampicillin-type drug or one of the nonsteroidal anti-inflammatory or antipyretic agents.

Table 2

Distinction between viral exanthemata and drug eruptions

	Viral eruptions	*Drug eruptions*
Epidemiological criterion	Yes, sometimes	No
General symptoms	Yes, usually	Mostly absent
Recurrences	No	Yes, sometimes
Drug challenge	Negative	Positive

Figure 89 Scarletiniform rash at different stages in brothers.

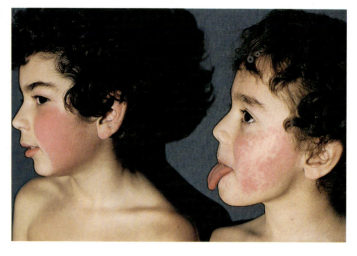

It should be noted that the above are diagnostic hints rather than absolute rules. Of more diagnostic value is a drug challenge test after resolution of the original eruption. In this test the suspected drug, in a tenth to a half of the usual dose, is administered to the subject while still in hospital. If the same rash occurs within twenty-four hours of administration this is excellent evidence incriminating the drug in question. Where there is some doubt, a full dose should be administered on a subsequent occasion. This simple test, when performed by experienced staff with the patient in hospital, carries very little risk and serves to incriminate or absolve a particular drug as the aetiological agent. The majority of roseola-like rashes are in fact viral in origin with members of the Coxsackie and echo groups being mainly responsible (Figures 90, 91).

Figure 90 Scarletiniform eruption caused by the echo virus. Note the raspberry-like appearance of the tongue and sheeted desquamation of the hands.

Figure 91 Scarletiniform eruption caused by Coxsackie virus. Note the striking desquamation.

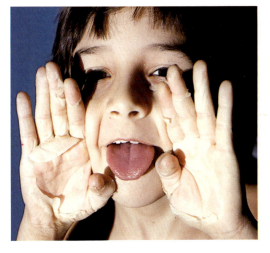

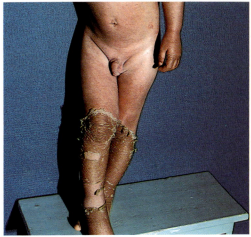

Erythma multiforme

This may be a type of vasculitis of the same general type as anaphylactic purpura and erythema nodosum and which is secondary to a provoking antigenic stimulus. Viral infection is often the preceipitating cause. Drugs, such as sulphonamides and non-steroidal anti-inflammatory agents, can also cause a similar disorder. EM is characterized by a peripheral distribution, i.e. the hands, feet, face. The primary lesion (Figure 92) is a papule with central exudation which enlarges peripherally, giving rise to a well-defined annular or target-shaped lesion.

It often is a recurrent disorder with fresh attacks occurring each autumn and spring, and can be an unpleasantly severe complaint. The mucosae are often involved – particularly the anterior mouth and the lips.

Treatment This is usually symptomatic, with cooling lotions and mouthwashes, but severely affected patients may require systemic steroids.

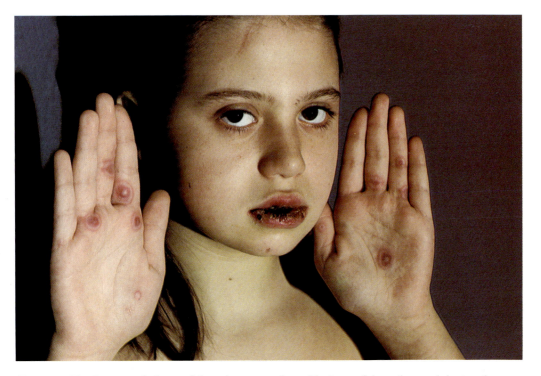

Figure 92 Erythema multiforme. Note the target-shaped lesions of the palms and the involvement of the lips.

Infantile papular acrodermatitis (Gianotti-Crosti syndrome)

This fairly uncommon disorder is distinguished by its association with hepatitis B. Typically the disorder is of sudden onset and without systemic disturbance. The rash is distributed primarily at the periphery, being most dense over the limbs and face, mostly avoiding the trunk. Large numbers of uniform erythematous papular lesions appear, some of which are purpuric (Figure 94).

Figure 93 Gianotti-Crosti syndrome.

Figure 94 Purpuric lesions of Gianotti-Crosti syndrome, caused by a rubber band.

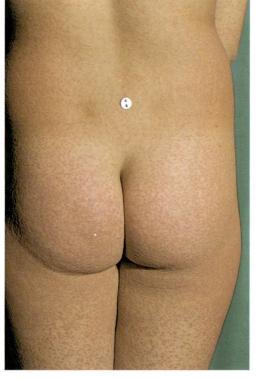

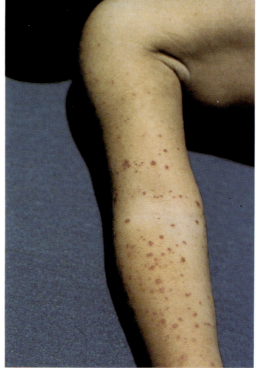

The appearance of the lesions should prompt the physician to perform liver function tests on the patient as characteristically the transaminases are found to be raised in this disorder. In addition, blood from the affected individuals will be Australia antigen positive. Usually the hepatitis is mild and jaundice does not occur, although, occasionally, the hepatitis is severe and proceeds to cirrhosis. The skin lesions persist for some three weeks and then disappear without trace. The differential diagnosis includes anaphylactoid purpura and peripherally distributed papular rashes. However, this disorder evolves in its own characteristic fashion and has its own distinctive clinical appearances. Furthermore, liver tests are normal in anaphylactic purpura.

Treatment   The Gianotti-Crosti syndrome is treated symptomatically.

Occasionally similar lesions occur without the characteristic peripheral distribution in the course of hepatitis B or another form of viral hepatitis.

Figure 95 Erythema multiforme-like lesions in a patient with anicteric hepatitis B.

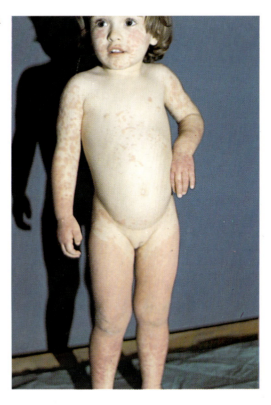

Fungus infections of skin

These are infections with micro-organisms derived from the vegetable kingdom which have lost the ability to synthesize chlorophyll. Dermatophyte fungi are weak pathogens that live in the stratum corneum. Primary fungal infection of skin is common and an important part of dermatological practice. Secondary infection with fungal micro-organisms, such as occurs in napkin dermatitis secondarily infected with candida albicans, should not be regarded as a true fungal infection.

The presence of dermatophytes can be demonstrated by examination of scale or skin scrapings or other preparations of stratum corneum or nail clippings. Mycelial filaments or rounded spores can be found in the infected horn or nail, depending on the particular infecting micro-organism. However, the micro-organism can only be correctly identified after culture in a selective medium, for example, Sabouraud's agar. Identification of the fungus after culture is based on the macroscopic appearance of the colonies and the metabolic capabilities of the cultured micro-organism.

This group of disorders is divided into dermatophyte infections (tinea, skin, nail and scalp infections), candidal and pityrosporon ovale infections and the deep fungus infections which are less common in the temperate climates of Europe.

Dermatophyte infections

There are superficial fungus infections of the skin, the most common of which in childhood is infection due to microsporum canis, which also infects cats and dogs. Interestingly, infection of the scalp with this fungus is restricted to children. Ringworm of the body, which is quite contagious, presents as small, scaling, red patches. Characteristically the affected areas enlarge rapidly to form eventually ring-like lesions (tinea, ringworm) (Figure 96). The coalescence of several of the affected areas causes the appearance of polycyclic lesions (Figure 97).

Treatment   In the mangement of ringworm infections the source of the infecting micro-organism should be sought and if possible eliminated. Treatment of individual lesions is now based on topical preparations of potent antimycotic drugs, including drugs of the imidazole type such as clotrimazole, miconazole and econazole and others such as tolnaftate. Systemic treatment is indicated in patients with severe widespread infection. Griseofulvin is only active against ringworm species (not candida albicans or pityrosporon ovale) and is prescribed in a dose of 15–20 mg/kg per day for fifteen to twenty days. Ketoconazole – another newer imidazole – is also useful and is prescribed in a dose of 5 mg/kg per day for fifteen to twenty days especially for severe candida infections.

Figure 96 Dermatophyte infection of the glabrous skin in mother and daughter. Note the regular, small, round red lesions.

Figure 97 Fungus infection of galbrous skin resulting in a polycyclic lesion.

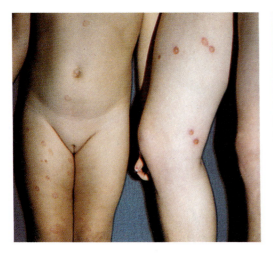

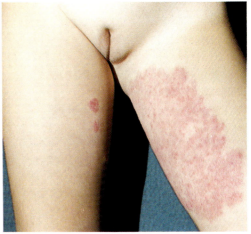

Ringworm of the scalp (tinea capitis)

Ringworm of the scalp can be divided into non-inflammatory and inflammatory (kerion) varieties. The non-inflammatory type, due to trichophyton species of fungus, causes perifollicular lesions and breaking of the hair shafts at the level of the scalp surface or 1–2 mm above the surface, resulting in a bald area (Figures 98, 99). On the bald areas, which are often multiple, minute 'black dots' due to broken hair shafts can be seen. Not all hairs are involved in the affected sites and some normal hair shafts are also present. Microscopic examination of affected hairs reveals large numbers of clusters of spores.

Figure 98 Scalp ringworm due to trichophyton infection. The differential diagnosis also includes alopecia areata in which there are no signs of terminal hair and inflammatory and scaling dermatoses of the scalp in which there are hairs of normal length (page 145).

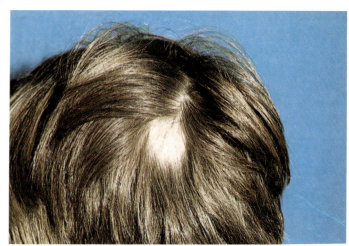

Microsporon infections are more frequent and contagious than those due to trichophyton species and often occur in small epidemics in schools – especially in deprived areas where levels of hygiene leave something to be desired. Microsporon infections of the scalp present as one quite large bald area (Figure 99). Sometimes ringworm lesions of the glabrous skin occur elsewhere simultaneously. Hairs generally break at a higher level than for trichophyton infection and microscopic examination of these broken hairs shows a mycelial network within the hair and small spores around the same hair shaft. Examination of the scalp in Wood's light (long wave ultraviolet light) will often reveal a dull greenish fluorescence in the affected area.

The diagnosis of tinea capitis is based on the presence of broken hairs set on an area of scaling scalp skin. The differential diagnosis includes trichotillomania (see page 98) but in this disorder the broken hairs are of variable length and there is no scaling of the scalp skin (Figure 98).

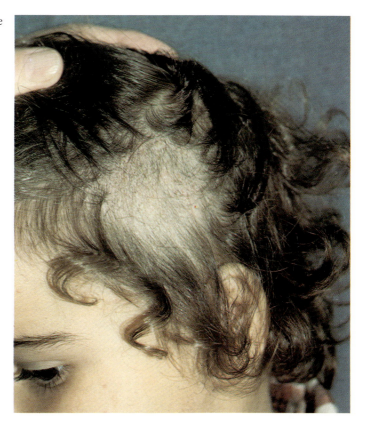

Figure 99 Scalp ringworm due to microsporon infection.

Treatment   The treatment of tinea capitis is based on administration of griseofulvin, 15–20 mg/kg per day for up to forty days. It is also prudent to cut the hair to 1 cm around the affected areas and then to apply one of the topical antimycotic preparations (one of the imidazole group of agents) daily.

Before the advent of griseofulvin the management of scalp ringworm presented a major problem. The affected children were contagious and their activities were curtailed accordingly. Because of this, various techniques for depilation were used in the past, including 'chemo-depilation' with thallium and X-irradiation. Both of these were responsible for unpleasant sequelae due to thallium toxicity and X-ray induced skin cancer.

Favus

Favus is the rarest of the dermatophye infections and has its own particular characteristics. It is the only fungus infection of the scalp that can strike at any time of life. The other forms of scalp ringworm are largely confined to prepubescent schoolchildren. Before the advent of griseofulvin these commoner forms of scalp ringworm in children spontaneously cleared at puberty and this has been supposed to be due to the antimycotic action of the fatty acid constituents of sebum that greatly increases in rate of secretion at the time of puberty.

Initially favus does not cause much in the way of hair loss because the invading fungal micro-organism does not result in breakage of the hair shafts. Affected areas seem to be dusted with a yellowish scale of dust from the profusion of fungal hyphae and spores.Many years later scarring alopecia may follow this disorder. Microscopically the parasitized hair may appear to have a double image due to the fungal hyphal mycelium. The differential diagnosis is in the main from a pyoderma of the scalp secondary to pediculosis, but microscopy of hairs from the affected area distinguishes the two conditions easily.

Treatment   This is the same as for ordinary scalp ringworm.

Figure 100 Favus. Note the yellowish, powdery appearance of the hairs in the involved area.

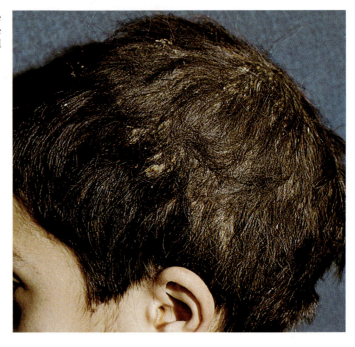

The invading dermatophyte fungi do not usually pass the dermo-epidermal barrier, so that marked inflammation is rare. When deeper invasion does occur, inflammatory ringworm results and on the scalp a kerion forms. Inflammatory ringworm clears spontaneously, and before griseofulvin was the only form of scalp ringworm to do so before puberty. Kerion results in scarring and there is permanent loss of hair in the scarred area. Clinically kerion usually presents as an inflamed, exuding and crusted nodule (Figure 101). The differential diagnosis includes other acute inflammatory disorders of the scalp, but microscopy of the hair and of the exudate should allow the correct diagnosis to be made.

Treatment   This is both local and systemic. Griseofulvin should be given systemically as for the other types of scalp fungus infection. In addition, local bathing with mild antiseptic lotions is recommended.

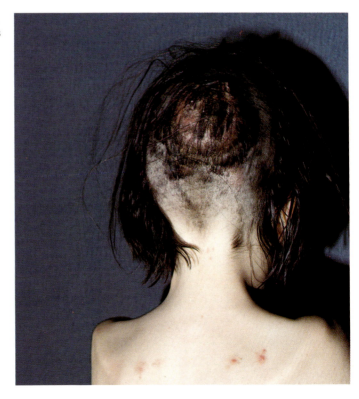

Figure 101 Kerion of the scalp. The hair around the lesion has been cut.

Candidiasis

Cutaneous candidiasis is caused in the majority of cases by the yeast candida albicans. It can exist either as spores or in a hyphal form, the latter being found in invaded tisue alongside the spore forms. The micro-organism parasitizes the superficial stratum corneum and mostly infects the body folds, the nails and mucosae of the buccal cavity, the anus and the vagina. It is often found in these sites as a saprophyte and only becomes invasive and pathogenic when the immune defences are in some way compromised as in prematurity, diabetes, AIDS, lymphoproliferative disorders and treatment with immunosuppressive agents. A common variety of candidiasis is oral thrush (Figure 102) in the second week of life, following infection contracted in passage through the vagina. Inguinal candidiasis is the most frequently involved flexural area in premature neonates and debilitated subjects but other areas can be involved (Figure 103).

Figure 102 Thrush in neonate in second week of life.

Figure 103 Candidiasis of interdigital skin in a baby.

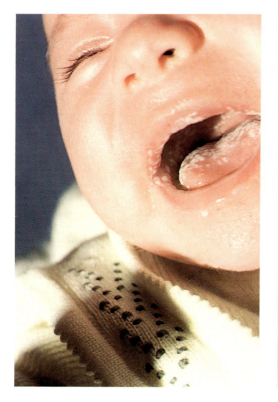

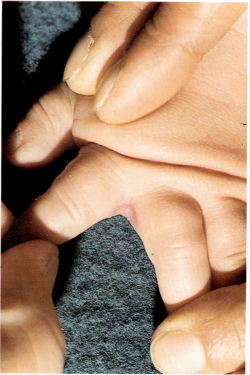

Chronic mucocutaneous candidiasis syndrome has several causes. It may be familial and is often the result of immunodeficiency. It often begins in the first year of life and may present as severe oral candidiasis or intractable onychomycosis (Figures 104, 105).

Treatment In mild disease the topical application of one of the imidazole group of drugs, or nystatin is usually rapidly successful. In chronic mucocutaneous candidiasis, systemic 5-flourocytosine has been used in some patients, but ketoconazole appears more useful.

Figure 104 Chronic mucocutaneous candidiasis involving the finger nails with severe deformity.

Figure 105 The same child as illustrated in Figure 104 after one year's treatment with ketoconazole.

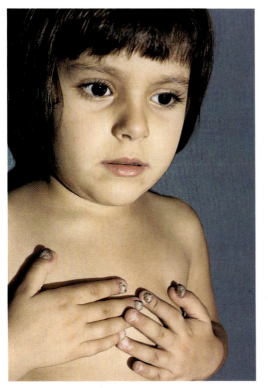

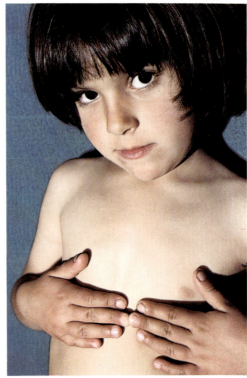

Cutaneous leishmaniasis

This is common in the Mediterranean basin, as well as being seen in many areas of Italy. The disease is caused by a protozoan micro-organism – leishmania tropica. The micro-organism is injected into the skin by the puncture of the bite of the sandfly (phlebotomus papatasii). The signs are variable. It varies from presenting as a small nodule to grave generalized disease.

The commonest form is the nodule which is rose-pink in colour. Later the nodule develops scaling centrally or becomes necrotic in its centre and develops an exudative surface which forms a crust. The face is commonly involved (Figure 106). Other exposed areas may also become involved.

The lupoid form is less frequently seen (Figure 107). It presents as a

Figure 106 Nodular leishmaniasis of forehead.　　**Figure 107** Lupoid leishmaniasis of face.

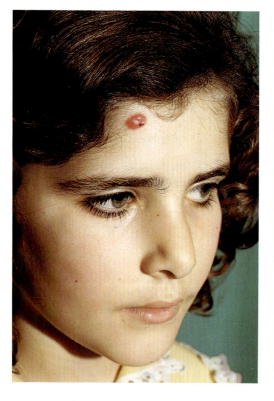

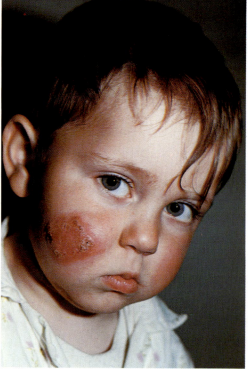

flattened, broad-based nodule of a dark red-brown colour on an exposed site. The diagnosis of the disease is based on its clinical features. In doubtful cases the diagnosis can be confirmed by biopsy and detection of the characteristic histological features (Figure 108). Rounded bodies with two different sized nuclei may be found.

Treatment The treatment of cutaneous leishmaniasis is based on antimonials such as stibogluconate. Because of the potential hepatic and renal toxicity of stilbogluconate, intralesional injection rather than systemic treatment by the intramuscular route is recommended.

Figure 108 Leishmania tropica in a smear from cutaneous leishmaniasis.

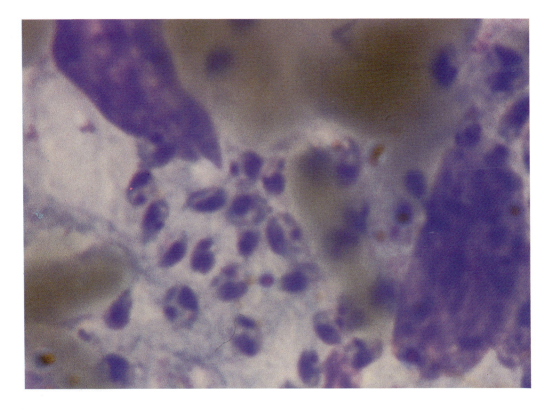

Scabies

Scabies is always a fairly common disorder although the prevalence varies from time to time, reaching epidemic proportions on occasion. The disease has become somewhat less common since 1976.

Scabies is caused by a mite – sarcoptes scabiei – which is an obligatory parasite on man alone. Transmission is therefore only by human contact. Infection is usually the result of prolonged bodily contact and therefore is often the result of sexual activity. However, this is not always the case, and it appears that the mite can be transmitted by more trivial types of contact.

Figure 109 A scabies burrow.

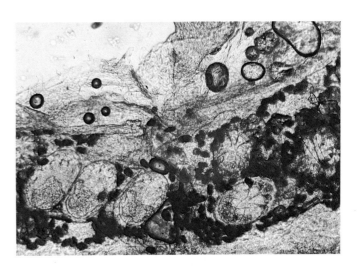

The fertilized female mite (Figure 109) excavates a tunnel in the more superficial layers of the stratum corneum in which she deposites her eggs. After some weeks the eggs hatch and nymphoid forms of the mite emerge. The scabies mite has similarities to the house dust mite (dermatophagoides) to which many atopic children are sensitized. It appears that some of the clinical signs of scabies, such as the nodules, are the result of hypersensitivity to the mite and/or its products, bearing a resemblance to a form of prurigo in children (papular urticaria).

The disorder is more frequent in socially deprived groups and may affect all members of a family and last for long periods. In temperate climates the disorder seems less common in the summer time and more frequent during school terms. Scabies may occur as early as the second week of life and has particular clinical appearances in the neonate. Itching is a prominent feature clinically but children scratch less frequently and this influences the appearance of the disorder.

Signs and symptoms   Scabies, papular urticaria and atopic dermatitis are the three most common itching skin disorders in children. The burrows caused by the female mite are pathognomonic of scabies. These are linear, or arciform, and are comma shaped. They are usually 1 mm wide and about 7 to 10 mm long. The presence of scratch marks is also important (but is less frequent in young children). Other typical, but not very common, lesions are pearly or whitish vesicles. These may be numerous and are found at the extremities of a burrow. More commonly found are papulovesicles (Figure 110) and nodules (Figure 111).

Figure 110 Scabies in a baby. Note the major concentration of the lesions around the axillae.

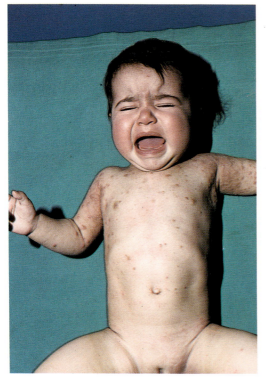

Figure 111 Typical nodular lesions in the axillary region.

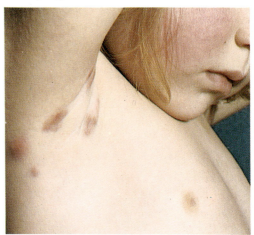

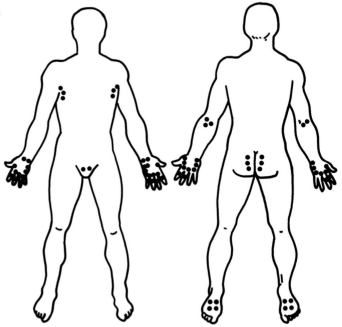

Diagram 1 Sites of predilection of scabies.

The distribution of lesions is of major diagnostic importance as the sites of predilection are typical and consistent. The main involved sites are the interdigital spaces, the ulnar border of the hand, the wrist flexures, over the elbows, the anterior axillary folds, the buttocks and the genitalia (see Diagram 1). In the first year of life the plantar aspects of the feet, and in the first month of life only, the head and neck, may also be involved. After treatment the lesions regress in a few weeks if there are no complications.

However, an attack of scabies does not confer lasting immunity. Nodular lesions are the last to disappear and may persist as red lumps for months, causing intense itching even though the mite has been eliminated and no further treatment is indicated.

Complications These are more frequent and more important in children. Infection is the most frequent complication and due to scratching. Impetiginization of the lesions is not uncommon and as a consequence of this, lymphangitis and lymphadenitis may arise (Figure 112). Glomerulonephritis may occur as a result of the secondary infection of the skin and in some geographical areas this has occurred in up to 10 per cent of patients with scabies.

Eczematization is a frequent complication in young children (Figure 113). This may involve large areas of the skin surface with papules, papulovesicles, scaling, erythema and exudation. The affected child may be extremely unwell and growth arrest during the illness is not uncommon.

Norwegian scabies is a variant of ordinary scabies found in the debilitated, in those with neurological disturbance or the mentally handicapped. This form of scabies (Figure 114, 115) is characterized by massive numbers of burrows that may cover the entire integument. On

Figure 112 Suppurative bacterial lymphandenitis in a child one year old due to scabies.

Figure 113 Post-scabetic eczema in a young child. Diffuse exudative erythematous lesions.

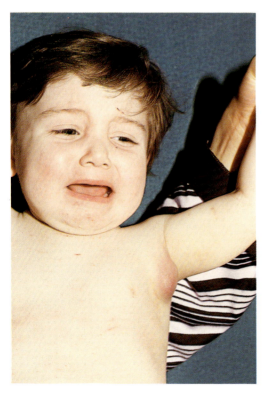

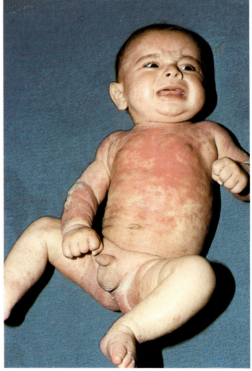

the palms and soles there may be gross hyperkeratosis (Figure 114) in which there are myriads of scabies mites. Norwegian scabies is amongst the most contagious of dermatological disorders.

Diagnosis This is based on the presence of burrows and the finding of the scabies mite in lesions. The mite can be obtained from scrapings of the skin surface obtained with a blunt scalpel blade or with a needle used to lay

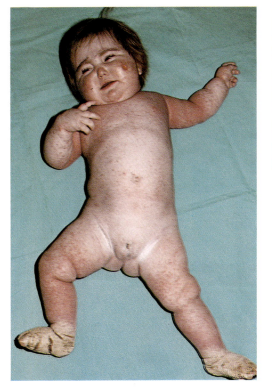

Figure 114 Norwegian scabies in a child of one year. Note the plantar hyperkeratosis.

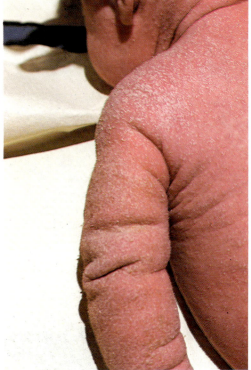

Figure 115 Norwegian scabies in a baby. Every one of the whitish lesions is a burrow.

open the burrow and spike the mite at its end. Scrapings of skin or material is transferred to a microscope slide and is examined microscopically for the presence of the mite, its eggs or faeces (Figure 109).

It is important that the disorder is looked for in other members of the family or household and in close friends. In particular the presence of itching in family and friends should be enquired after. Of course other causes of itching should be borne in mind, but if there is itchiness of an individual who may have had close contact with the patient and this has arisen at approximately the same time, then scabies should be suspected. It should be remembered that papular urticaria and atopic dermatitis are remittent and persistent disorders.

Differential diagnosis Infantile lichenoid acrodermatitis may be considered in the differential diagnosis but of course no mites will be found in scrapings of the affected areas in this disorder and there are no burrows. Mastocytosis may be considered in the differential diagnosis of nodular scabies.

Treatment Gammexane- and benzyl benzoate- containing lotions are both effective. All the body surface should be treated (apart from the head and neck) after a hot bath. It is usual to give a second painting with the medicament some twenty-four hours after the first treatment. Some dermatologists recommend a third application approximately seven days later.

In children of less than two years old, great care should be taken, as both gammexane and benzyl benzoate are irritants. For these youngsters 5 per cent sulphur (sulfur) in cream may be less irritating.

It is important that the treatment is used on all the body areas as advised, and not just applied to the obviously involved sites. For this reason it is usual to supply printed instructions with the medicaments. It is also important that other members of the household, and close friends, are treated at the same time.

In the first year of life the head and neck should be included in the treatment regime. If a sulphur preparation is used it is best to apply this for three to five successive evenings without bathing before application. Although the mite does not live in the clothes it is prudent to have these washed. Disinfection of the house is not required. In nodular scabies, after the specific treatments detailed above, it is useful to recommend treatment as for atopic dermatitis with a corticosteroid-containing topical application. It should be noted that the irritant nature of the specific miticidal agents often prolongs the eczematization. This may lead the affected individual to believe that he or she is still infected with the scabies mite and to apply more of the irritant material. For this reason it is useful also to supply a bland antipruritic material such as oily calamine for use after the specific treatment.

Tick bites

It is important to remember that tick bites can cause headaches in children and, in the most severely affected individuals, are responsible for encephalitis. They are usually seen on the heads of children that play with dogs, or who live in the country and enjoy playing on the ground. Although the diagnosis is easy for the experienced observer, it is not unusual for children to present in the clinic with the tick still attached to the scalp with the mistaken diagnosis of wart or papilloma. In such patients the lesions may be quite necrotic (Figures 116, 117).

Treatment   The ticks can be removed by inserting a forceps between the tick head and the skin and gently forcing the tick out of the skin.

Figure 116 Necrotic area from a tick bite.

Figure 117 Ulcerated area due to necrotic tick bite.

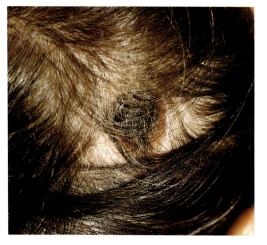

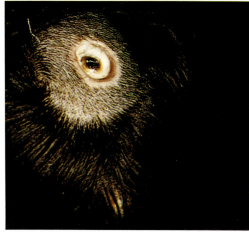

Papular urticaria

This disorder is caused by hypersensitivity to antigenic material of biting arthropods in predisposed individuals. Presumably the irritant substances or the antigens are introduced by the bites or stings of the insects responsible. Clearly lesions at the site of bites occur in all individuals attacked by insects. However, allergic mechanisms are responsible for lesions occurring elsewhere in predisposed subjects. There can be little doubt that the above mechanism is at the root of the pathogenesis of papular urticaria, although many other mechanisms have been proposed.

Figure 118 Insect bites.

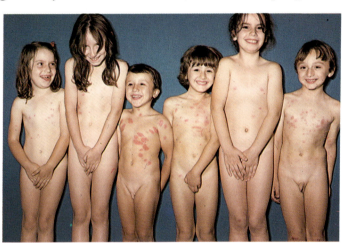

The disorder has a seasonal predilection and presumably this is supportive of the hypersensitivity mechanism stated. The reason for the predisposition is unclear, but some of the patients are atopics, as evidenced by the raised IgE levels in many subjects.

Affected individuals are usually two to seven years of age. In very young children, lesions may be very extensive (Figure 121). The lesions occur in the summer months (May to August) and tend to recur annually at the same time for some years. They appear mainly in the exposed sites of face and limbs, reflecting the sites of insect bites, and often start with large blisters (Figure 119) or oedematous swellings (Figure 121) which are intensely irritant. After a period that varies from a few hours to some days, the erythematous halo disappears and the central papulovesicular region remains. This lesion lasts some ten to fifteen days in all but may become intermittently more inflamed before finally disappearing. Recrudescence of the lesion may occur if there is a bite at another site. A pigmented area may remain after all the inflammatory swelling has subsided.

Treatment   This is based on understanding the life cycle of the parasite responsible. When the mosquito causes the disorder every effort should be made to prevent the child being bitten by these insects. Frequent use of insect repellents on exposed skin sites is indicated during the day and prevention of mosquitoes from entering the bedroom at night is also prudent.

The itch from the disorder may be treated by topical applications such as mentholated oily calamine lotion or 1 per cent hydrocortisone cream. Local antihistamine preparations are ineffectual and may cause allergic sensitization, but systemic antihistamines may give some relief.

Figure 119 Bullous papular urticaria.

Figure 121 Profuse lesions of papular urticaria in a baby.

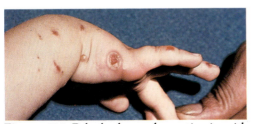

Figure 120 Palpebral papular urticaria with marked oedema.

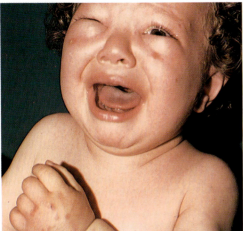

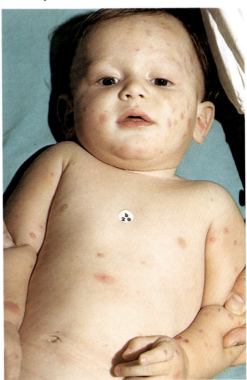

Burns

Burns of all kinds are more frequent in childhood (Figures 122, 123) because of the comparative lack of responsibility of children and sometimes their parents.

Treatment In grade 1 burns, characterized by oedema and erythema, only treatment with topical hydrocortisone preparations may help to reduce the inflammation and pain.

The treatment of the more severe grade 2 or grade 3 burns is more complex and dependent on the extent of the burn. With localized lesions, any blister roofs should be punctured and the area bathed frequently with hypochlorite solution. Necrotic tissue should be removed and the areas treated with an antibacterial application – silver sulphadiazine has been shown to be quite effective.

It is important to follow patients who have been burnt quite closely in order to treat any unsightly scarring (Figure 123) as soon as possible. Exuberant granulation tissue may be treated with silver nitrate sticks. Once keloid scarring has been established there is little that can be done.

Figure 122 Burns from fireworks carried in the pocket.

Figure 123 Keloids from burns.

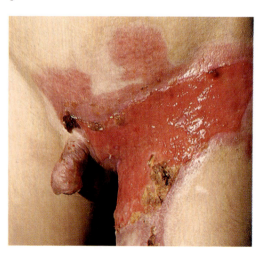

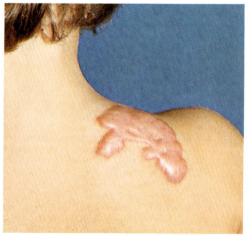

Photodermatitis

The lesions of a photodermatitis follow exposure to solar ultraviolet light or, more uncommonly, exposure to ultraviolet light (UVL) from an artificial source (Figure 124). It is believed that either of two mechanisms may be involved – either phototoxicity or photoallergy. In phototoxicity the reaction is due to enhancement of the toxic properties of a substance by UVL, so that it becomes allergenic.

Among the substances frequently responsible must be numbered oil of bergamot. This fragrance, derived from bergamot fruit, contains 5-methoxypsoralen which causes phototoxicity. Oil of bergamot has been included in numerous toiletry articles, including those used for children. Exposure to the sun after use of one of the applications containing oil of bergamot may provoke a dermatitis that is followed by pigmentation that may take many years to resolve.

Figure 124 Extensive photodermatitis and keratitis from ultraviolet light.

Figure 125 Photodermatitis from oil of bergamot in a perfume.

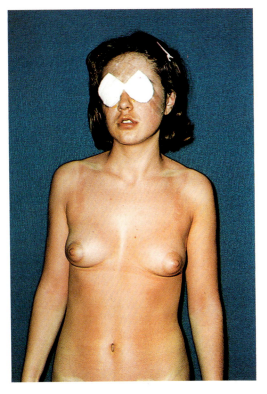

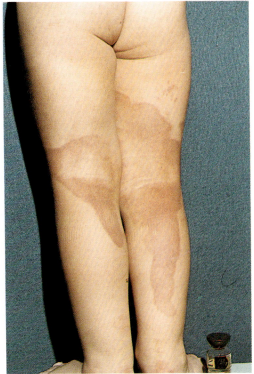

Sweat rashes (sudamina, miliaria)

Sweat rashes are most common in babies under two years old and are provoked by all the stimuli that cause a rise in body temperature. Some individuals appear to be predisposed to the problem and this may explain why the condition may last as long as four to five months in the warm season.

The degree and site of obstruction of the sweat glands and the amount of inflammation present determine the clinical picture. The picture varies from the uninflamed miliaria crystallina, in which numerous whitish vesicles are clustered together (but not coalescing) at the site of skin contact with clothing, to miliaria rubra (Figure 126) in which the typical lesions are rose-red papulovesicles, and to miliaria profunda, in which there are larger dark papules and nodules. The last type is rare in European climates.

Treatment   This consists of reducing the body temperature and using general local and systemic measures to relieve the symptoms. It should be noted that topical corticosteroids and antihistamines are of little value. In severely affected subjects it may be necessary to transfer the child to a cooler environment.

Figure 126 Miliaria rubra with numerous uniform papulovesicles.

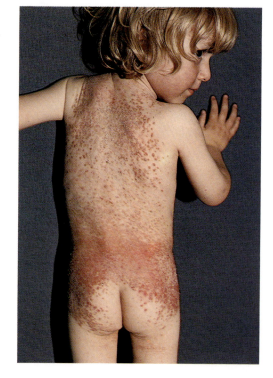

Napkin dermatitis

Napkin dermatitis is one of the most frequent problems in the first two years of life.

Aetiology   Napkins are quite obviously important in the cause of this disorder, as it can be seen to be distributed over the convexities of the buttocks, with sparing of the creases and folds (Figure 127). A similar condition may occur in older children (Figure 128) or adults who for some reason have to return to wearing napkins. The effects of close contact of stagnant urine and faeces with the skin under the napkin is aggravated by

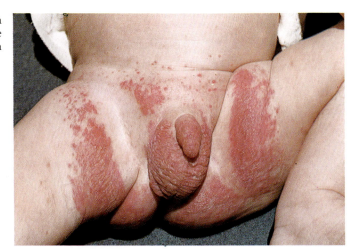

Figure 127 Typical napkin dermatitis with sparing of the flexures and accentuation on the convexities.

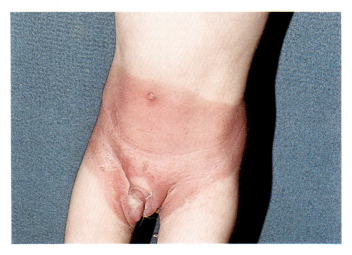

Figure 128 Napkin dermatitis in an incontinent child of four. Note the line of demarcation caused by the edge of the plastic pants.

the maceration of the napkin area caused by the wearing of plastic pants.

Secondary infection of the skin damaged in the way described, with a variety of bacteria, including staphylococci as well as by candida albicans, may play some role in the clinical picture. Such infections resolve spontaneously with the need for antimicrobial measures when the contact with urine and faeces is stopped and the condition starts to improve. These secondary invaders may be a particular problem in the depths of the skin folds especially in the debilitated or premature child.

Symptomatology The lesions are localized to the convexities of the buttocks and pubis (Figure 127). The morphology of the rash itself is variable and is not indicative of the causative agent. However, aggregated whitish pustules may be indicative of candida albicans superinfection.

In the majority of cases napkin dermatitis has the appearance of an irritant contact dermatitis in which there are confluent, intensely congested and sometimes exudative erythematous areas (Figure 131). When the affected areas are isolated they may have a different morphology with either papular lesions (Figure 132) or pustular lesions (Figure 133) predominating. When the inflammatory stimulus is very vigorous,

Figure 129 Micropustular lesions of candida albicans.

Figure 130 Close up of Figure 129, showing pustules and scalloped desquamation.

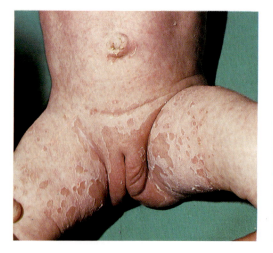
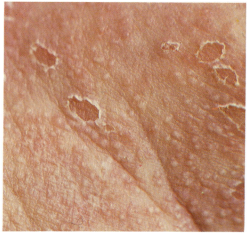

ulcerative lesions (Figure 134) and gangrenous lesions (Figure 135) may be present.

Natural history Napkin dermatitis is rarely an isolated incident. Generally, recurrences are provoked by infrequent changes of napkin, episodes of diarrhoea, and drug administration (particularly antibiotics).

Figure 131 Erythematous confluent lesions of the irritative type.

Figure 132 Napkin dermatitis with papular lesions.

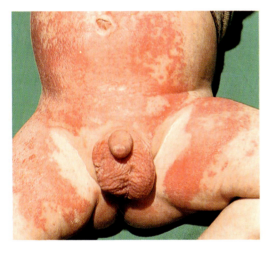

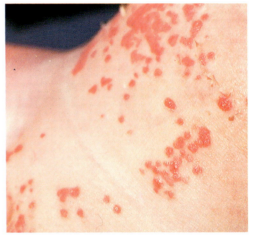

Figure 133 Napkin dermatitis with pustular lesions.

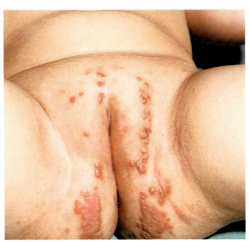

Figure 134 Napkin dermatitis with ulcerative lesions.

Figure 135 Necrotic lesions due to the presence of a caustic substance accidentally present in the napkin.

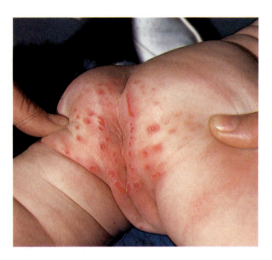
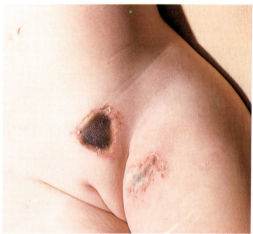

The tendency to relapse disappears when napkins and plastic pants are no longer used.

Complications   In 15 per cent of children with napkin dermatitis, rashes occur on other sites. This generally happens some weeks or months after the start of the napkin dermatitis, in an explosive manner, with lesions occurring on the face and successively over the limbs and trunk. The secondary lesions are initially punctuate but then enlarge rapidly and become confluent, to affect much of the site involved. These peripheral lesions generally last no more than one to three months and then spontaneously remit. They do not tend to recur with future episodes of napkin rash. They may have a psoriasiform appearance (Figure 136) or a papulovesicular appearance and are more plainly eczematous (Figure 137). Although the spread may suggest an allergic contact hypersensitivity, tests for this do not support this mechanism.

Figure 136 Napkin dermatitis with secondary, psoriasiform eruption.

Figure 137 Napkin dermatitis with secondary eczematous eruption.

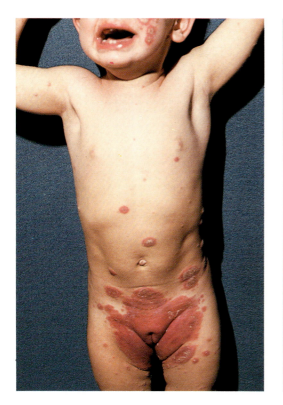

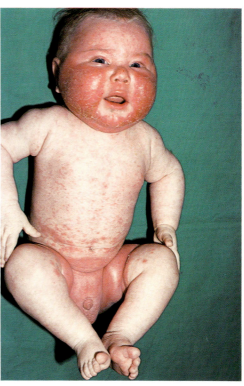

It is possible that the secondary spread of napkin rash (seen in 15 per cent of patients) is due to hypersensitivity to candidal antigens, in a similar way to that observed in the course of inguinal dermatophyte infection seen in the adult. However, the evidence for this is just as incomplete.

Other complications of napkin dermatitis are due in the main to inappropriate treatment – in particular topical corticosteroids. Gluteal granuloma is one unpleasant such complication. This occurs usually in children between four and nine months of age in the course of napkin dermatitis. Large, hard, well-defined plum- or violet-coloured nodules appear in the napkin area, causing alarm to the parents. The medical attendants who are generally unfamiliar with the problem because of its recent description tend also to be quite concerned about these lesions! The lesions persist for three to six weeks and are resistant to treatment. They disappear gradually, leaving atrophic scarring. As these lesions have only been recognized in the past twenty years or so it seems likely that

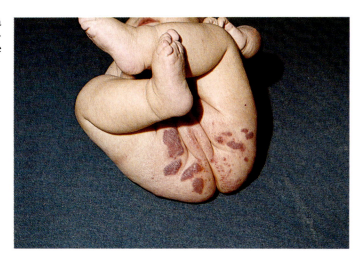

Figure 138 Gluteal granuloma in napkin dermatitis as a consequence of the prolonged use of a topical corticosteroid.

their appearance is bound up with the use of potent topical corticosteroids to the napkin area, where percutaneous penetration is enhanced because of the thinness of the skin, the occlusion of the napkin and the disturbed skin barrier function due to the dermatitis (Figure 138).

The differential diagnosis of napkin rashes is of considerable importance, as many disorders can localize in the inguino-anal region because of the vasodilatation in the area. Although some conditions are rare, their recognition is vital or else the life of the child may be endangered. Acrodermatitis enteropathica, caused by faulty zinc metabolism, is such a disorder (Figure 139). It often begins as a fiery eruption in the inguino-anal region as is associated with severe diarrhoea and alopecia. Congenital syphilis (Figure 140) may present as a papular eruption in the same region and if suspected, should be confirmed by serological tests. Histiocytosis X can also begin in the napkin area as small papular lesions (see page 136). These quickly become purpuric and are associated with hepatosplenomegaly and haematological disorders.

Two other skin conditions may mimic napkin dermatitis. These are seborrhoeic dermatitis and atopic dermatitis. Seborrhoeic dermatitis has a characteristic evolution. It usually begins in the first month of life and remits in the fourth month. The scalp and the root of the nose are affected by reddish-yellow scaling. Atopic dermatitis can be confused with napkin dermatitis when the latter is disseminated to other areas. The itching and a family history of the atopic state (allergic rhinitis, atopic dermatitis and asthma) should serve to distinguish atopic dermatitis. Another helpful feature is the presence of involvement of the deep folds of the inguinal

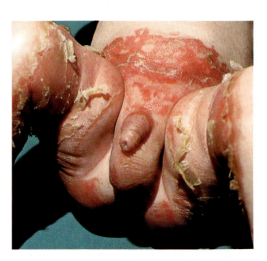

Figure 139 Acrodermatitis enteropathica with typical fiery, erosive lesions.

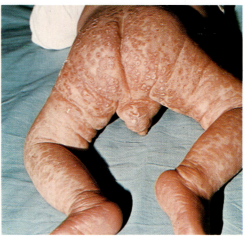

Figure 140 Congenital syphilis with papular lesions in the inguino-anal region.

region. Candidiasis of the flexures (Figure 141) is seen in debilitated and premature children, and is usually accompanied by oral candidiasis. Less commonly, sweat rashes and bullous impetigo will enter the differential diagnosis.

Treatment It is important to try to attack the cause of the disorder by greatly reducing the degree of contact with urine and faeces and by prohibiting occlusive garments such as plastic pants. Mothers should be told to change the napkin as soon as it is soiled, and preferably the napkin itself should be made of pure cotton. It may also be useful to suggest that after washing, the napkins are thoroughly rinsed. The affected skin should be washed without ordinary toilet soap, though emollient cleansing agents or oils may be used. After washing, the areas should be patted dry – not rubbed vigorously. In mildly affected infants these measures are usually sufficient.

Figure 141 Candidiasis of flexures in a premature baby.

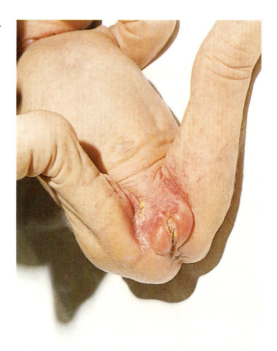

When there is much inflammation, the best treatment consists of compresses of physiological saline. Compresses of boric acid solution should not be used because of their potential toxicity. Compresses should be renewed whenever the napkin is changed. When the rash becomes less inflamed, a zinc cream may be used. When there is generalization of napkin dermatitis, hospitalization may be required.

In rashes which last longer than seventy-two hours, superinfection by candida albicans should be suspected and a topical anti-yeast cream, for example, nystatin, clotrimazole or econazole should be applied t.i.d. Antibiotics should be reserved for patients in whom there is a clear indication. Similarly, topical corticosteroids are needed infrequently, and should only be prescribed if really indicated, as they are readily absorbed and can lead to gluteal granuloma, iatrongenic Cushing's syndrome (Figure 142) and skin atrophy.

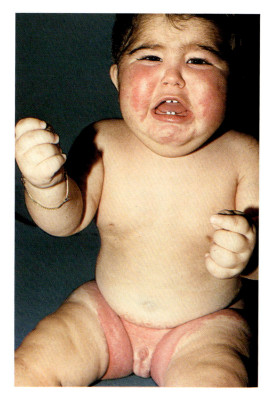

Figure 142 Cushing's syndrome from percutaneous absorption of topical corticosteroids used in the napkin area.

Factitial dermatitis (syn. dermatitis artefacta)

The term factitial dermatitis implies a skin disorder caused by the patients themselves or some other individual. In some cases the cause is frivolous, as in the patient portrayed in Figure 143, in which a glass was placed over the mouth, and the negative pressure from the suction applied caused a purpuric rash. In other cases habit tics are responsible, as for example, trichotillomania (Figure 144) or excoriated acne – syn, acné excorié (Figures 145, 146).

In trichotillomania, which generally occurs after the second year of life, the child usually twists the hair around the fingers and then tugs it in a

Figure 143 Purpura from suction due to application of a glass.

Figure 144 Trichotillomania. Note the regularity of the lesion and the presence of hairs of varying lengths.

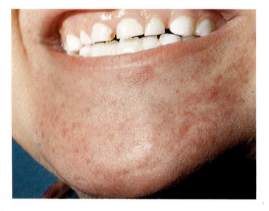

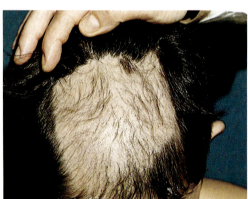

Figures 145 and 146 Excoriated acne lesions on the face and back of the hand due to repeated scratching.

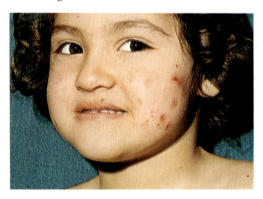

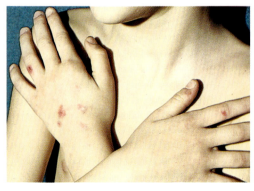

repetitive way – always in the same way and at the same site. This often results in a well-defined pattern of hair loss. The child's habit is usually evident when watching television, while falling asleep or when pre-occupied by daydreams. The different lengths of broken hair and the absence of signs of inflammation from the scalp are characteristic and permit the diagnosis.

In excoriated acne the lesions are generally localized to the face and may simulate true acne occurring postpubertally. It causes many small crusted and inflamed lesions to appear. The condition generally improves as the child matures, when the realization arrives that it is due to his or her own activities and results in an unaesthetic appearance. In some cases the intervention of a child psychiatrist can be useful.

Sometimes lesions are caused by one or another of the parents whose activities are unrecognized by the other spouse. The responsible parent may not admit their action because of all the social furore that it may cause.

Figure 147 Non-accidental injury in a child.

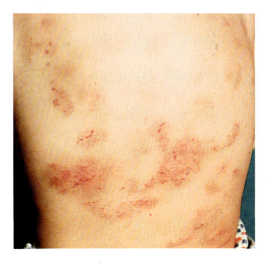

Atopic dermatitis

Atopic dermatitis is the skin disorder that, along with asthma and allergic rhinitis, is a manifestation of the atopic state. The atopic state may be regarded as a complex state of immunological and pharmocological disequilibrium.

Frequency and natural history Atopic dermatitis is an extremely common skin disorder of childhood. It has been calculated that approximately 3 per cent of pre-school children are affected by it. It is a chronic disorder that lasts for some years and even decades, causing considerable disturbance to the child and to those in close contact with it.

Relationship to asthma In about a quarter of cases of atopic dermatitis, the skin disorder precedes the development of asthma.

Cause Atopic dermatitis, or at least, the propensity to develop it, is a genetically determined disorder, although the mode of hereditary transmission is not clear. It seems that exogenous factors are also necessary to make the disorder manifest. The evidence for the genetic component to the disorder stems from the fact that 70 per cent of affected children have either a parent or a sibling who is affected by the same condition, or, less frequently, by other atopic disorders. Also in favour of its basically inherited nature is the finding of elevated levels of the

Figure 148 Atopic dermatitis in a four months old child and his mother.

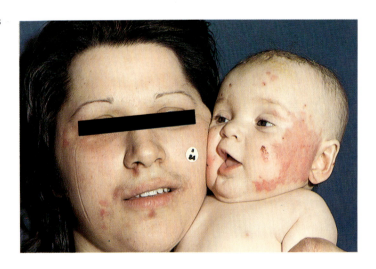

immunoglobulin IgE in the umbilical cord blood of neonates who are later affected by the disorder.

Elevated levels of IgE are characteristic of the atopic state and the extent of the increase mirrors the severity of the disorder. The finding of an increase in IgE levels in the blood is only one of the complex immunological alterations found in atopic dermatitis, as disorders of cell mediated immunity are also found. In particular there seems to be an abnormality of or deficit in the T-lymphocyte suppressor cells. The suppressor lymphocytes have the function of suppressing immuno-globulin production. The deficit in suppressor lymphocyte activity is more likely to be part of the genetically inherited fault and the elevated IgE levels may be secondary to this disorder of lymphocyte function.

Non-immunological factors also seem to play an important role. The characteristic dryness of the skin (Figure 149) has been believed by some to be in part due to alterations in the secretions of the sebaceous and sweat glands. However, others have reported that the dryness is in reality part of the eczematous process. Abnormal reactivity to certain pharmacological stimuli is also characteristic of atopic subjects. Stroking the skin of atopic patients firmly with a blunt object, for example, a knuckle or key, results in a white line (white dermographism) rather than the usual red-coloured

Figure 149 Dry skin on the arm of a boy with atopic dermatitis of the hands and elbows.

Figure 150 Atopic facies. Note characteristic facial pallor.

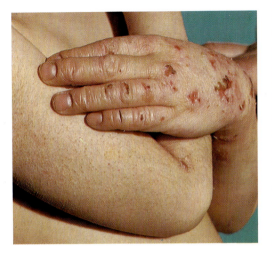

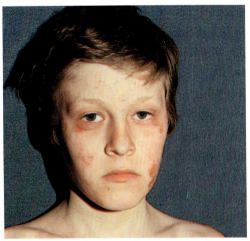

stripe. Pallor of the skin (Figure 150) is also typical of the atopic state.

The illness usually begins in the first months of life, concomitant with weaning. It is for this reason that some authorities believe that dietary factors play some role in the development of the disorder. Cow's milk and eggs are the most incriminated. Skin tests and tests for the presence of specific IgE antibodies do indicate that in atopic dermatitis there is a high degree of immunoreactivity to these foodstuffs. Despite this there is little real evidence that either cow's milk or eggs actually cause the disorder. Dietary treatment of atopic dermatitis has fallen in and out of fashion for many years and it is sad that there is still no final answer to the question: does exclusion of these foods improve the disorder? Some children, especially in the first year of life, seem to be helped, but they are few and there is no way of predicting which these will be. Many who have an undeniable allergic response to eggs and milk lose their allergy after a few years, but their atopic dermatitis persists. Food allergies are generally of the immediate hypersensitivity type, causing urticaria and angioedema (Figures 151, 152), asthma and gastrointestinal symptoms due to fixation of the reaginic antibodies on mast cells in the skin and mucosae. Recent laboratory studies strongly suggest that the IgE antibodies to any of the dietary allergens are not involved in the pathogenesis of the dermatitis.

It should be stressed that in order to validate the causative role of any food or food component, it is necessary to demonstrate regression of the dermatitis after exclusion of the foodstuff, and relapse after its re-introduction. To add to the difficulties in the interpretation of the results of exclusion and challenge tests, it must be remembered that the disease is subject to spontaneous remission and relapse. The disorder also varies with the climate, worsening in the winter and spring and improving in the summer. In addition, the disorder can sometimes dramatically improve after hospitilization – even without any form of topical or systemic treatment. It may also improve quite spontaneously after a move to a new house.

Figures 151 and 152 Child with severe atopic dermatitis and an allergy to fish. A few mgs of fish provoked angioedema and urticaria after a few minutes. There was no aggravation of his eczema and there was no improvement when fish was excluded from the diet.

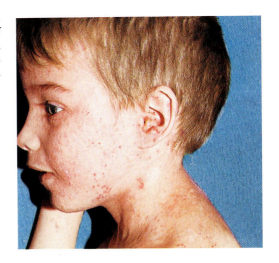

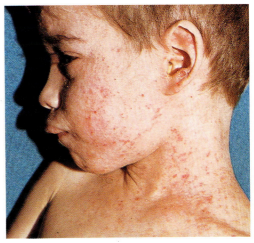

Symptoms   The symptoms are often less dramatic than in the adult. This is also true for other disorders such as herpes zoster and urticaria. However, this disorder, along with papular urticaria and scabies, does cause intense itching at times (Figures 153, 154). The itching is often precipitated by fluctuations in temperature. For example, itching is often intense after undressing, lying in bed, or during sweating after exercise. Trivial stimuli, for example, rough clothing made from wool or synthetic fibres, may also evoke intense itching. Some foods may provoke a perioral erythema in the atopic child via irritant and non-allergenic stimulation. These foods include tomatoes, citrus foods and cheeses.

The itching of atopic dermatitis provokes scratching after the third month. Before this time the child may cry and be irritable, as well as suffer from sleeplessness. The itching and consequent scratching results in

Figure 153 Intensely irritative impetiginized atopic dermatitis.

Figure 154 Generalized atopic dermatitis with intensely irritant atopic dermatitis.

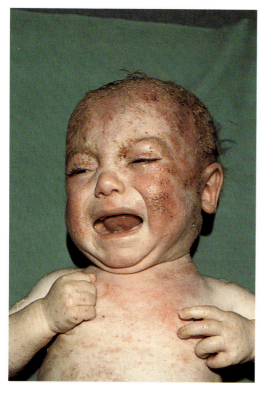

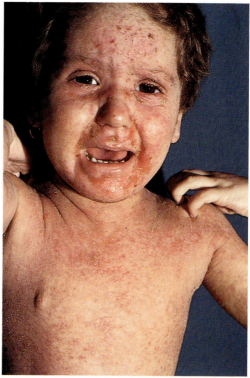

lichenification (lichenification is skin thickening with accentuation of skin markings).

The essential physical features of atopic dermatitis are erythema, vesiculation and scaling. The chronic lesions are lichenified. Usually there is erythema and scaling of the affected skin on a background of generalized roughness of the skin surface. In places there may be some vesiculation and exudation especially round the flexures. In the first year the lesions may be more intensely inflamed (Figure 156) with vesiculation or more usually exudation. The lesions themselves are in no way pathognomonic but the sites of involvement are helpful in diagnosis. Classically the flexor surfaces of the antecubital (Figure 157) and popliteal (Figure 158) fossae are involved symmetrically – a pattern of disease rarely seen in other

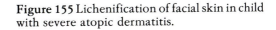

Figure 155 Lichenification of facial skin in child with severe atopic dermatitis.

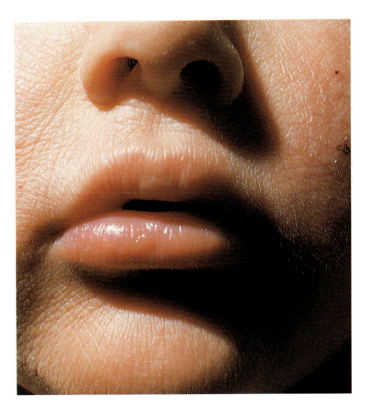

diseases. The other flexural areas are less often involved. If the head and neck are involved there is a characteristic involvement of the zygomatic regions. The skin around the eyes and mouth and under the ears (Figure 160) is also often affected. The hands and, to a lesser extent, the feet are often involved; the trunk is less frequently attacked.

The age of the patient seems to be important in determining the sites of involvement and the morphology of the lesions. In the first year of life the rash tends to be more inflamed and exudative. As the child ages, vesiculation is less frequently seen, and the lesions tend to be pink and

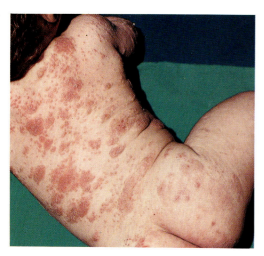

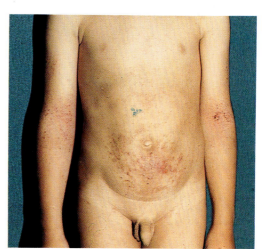

Figure 156 Diffuse erythematous exudative lesions in a child of nine months.

Figure 157 Typical lesions of atopic dermatitis in the antecubital fossae.

Figure 158 Typical lesions of atopic dermatitis in the popliteal fossae.

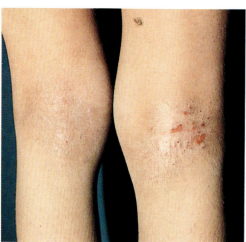

scaly. In the first few months the lesions can involve much of the skin surface and rarely cause an erythroderma. After this time the most important sites are, as mentioned previously, the antecubital and popliteal fossae. The involvement of hands may result in accentuation of the palmar creases, although this is more frequently seen in adults.

Complications   Impetiginization of the skin is not as frequently seen as might be expected, when it is realized that these patients' immunological defence mechanisms are impaired and the barrier function of their skin is also faulty. When it does occur it may be seen in the first few months of life and tends to recur later as well. Impetiginization is first obvious by increased exudation of the affected site. Later, pustules are seen, and are quickly followed by a yellowish-green crust and scale (Figures 161, 162).

Figure 159 In the first two years of life the zygomatic regions are involved with sparing of the central facial zone.

Figure 160 After the first two years of life, the areas around the eyes, the perioral region, and the skin under the ears, tend to be affected.

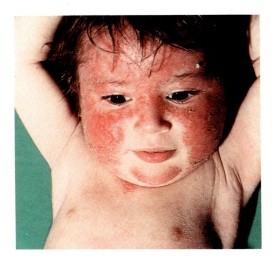

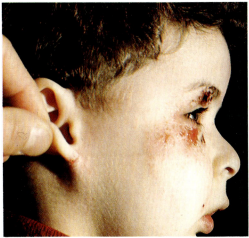

Viral infections of the skin are more frequent in atopic subjects. They are especially prone to infection with the herpes virus and to the vaccinia virus, although at the time of writing, vaccination is no longer routinely practised. Infections with papilloma viruses, causing warts, are also more frequent.

The most unpleasant complication is primary infection with herpes virus after contact with an individual with herpes simplex lesions. This mostly occurs towards the end of the first year of life after contact with a relative with recurrent cold sores. The onset is usually abrupt, with general malaise and fever. The eczematous areas are at first more inflamed and then become densely studded with vesiculopustules 1 to 2 mm in diameter, some of which are umbilicated. Although death may rarely occur, as may ocular complications and encephalitis, the disorder generally resolves spontaneously in approximately fifteen days and in general does not recur.

Allergic contact dermatitis may also complicate the disorder. This is rare in early infancy but more frequent in children after the age of six or seven years (Figure 164) in whom vesicular dermatitis of the hands and feet develops. The more common sensitizing agents are the dichromates and nickel, paraphenylenediamine (blue-black dyes) and constituents of topical treatments, including neomycin and sulphonamides (sulfona-mides). After contact with the particular sensitizer, the skin reacts with typical eczematous lesions.

Diagnosis This is straightforward when the disorder is persistent and occurs in the typical sites. It may be more difficult in the first few months of life when atopic dermatitis has to be differentiated from seborrhoeic dermatitis. When the clinical manifestations are not typical, other disorders, in which eczematoid disorders occur, must be borne in mind. These include phenylketonuria and the Wiskott-Aldrich syndrome.

As there are no pathognomonic clinical or laboratory findings in atopic dermatitis it is necessary to set up and adhere to criteria before making the diagnosis. The criteria are as follows: (1) pruritus, (2) lesions in typical sites, (3) a recurrent course that begins before the first year of life, (4) coexistence of other atopic manifestations such as asthma and allergic rhinitis and (5) the same disorder in parents or siblings. According to most authorities, three or more of these criteria should be satisfied if the diagnosis is to be established. In the first year of life, care must be taken to distinguish atopic dermatitis from seborrhoeic dermatitis and napkin dermatitis with spread. The diagnostic criteria are set out in the table below.

Figures 161 and 162 Impetiginized atopic dermatitis. The infection was not recognized and was treated with herbal remedies. In Figure 162 the child has received one day of antibiotic treatment.

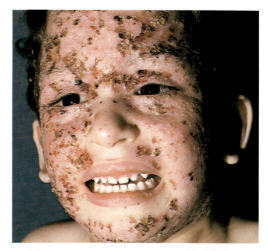

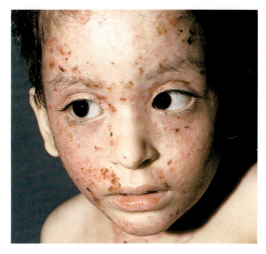

Laboratory investigations The value of the total IgE blood level is sometimes helpful in the diagnosis, although the total IgE is only raised in 60 to 70 per cent of patients with atopic dermatitis. It should also be remembered that IgE levels can be raised in other diseases, including scabies and papular urticaria – which are also itching dermatoses. The levels of IgE in the normal population vary considerably (5–300 iu/ml) and although the mean normal IgE level is less than the mean for patients with atopic dermatitis, there is considerable overlap. Raised IgE level may persist for some years after the disorder has subsided and stay elevated during quiescent phases of the disease. Furthermore, severe atopic dermatitis may present with normal or barely elevated IgE levels. For these reasons the IgE level cannot be used to follow the progress of atopic dermatitis.

The RAST test (radio-allergosorbent test) can be used to pinpoint to which of the environmental allergens there are IgE antibodies in the blood. However, it is easy to fall into the trap of believing that because

Figure 163 Herpetic infection on pre-existing atopic dermatitis of the face.

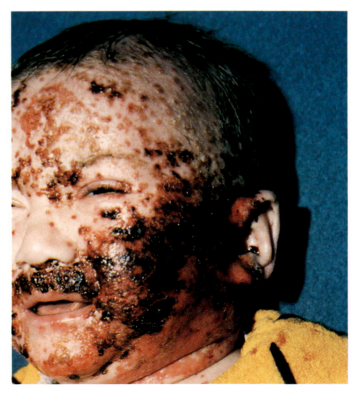

there are antibodies present they have significance for the pathogenesis of the disorder. This is by no means the case, and it is unjustifiable to start diets or other allergen avoidance manoeuvres without other evidence. This advice is supported by the negative results of numerous treatment trials based on the finding of antibodies to this or that antigen in the blood. The existence of such antibodies is probably no more than evidence that the individual has 'met' that particular antigen and has a heightened ability to make IgE antibodies. Before attributing a role to an antigen incriminated in the RAST test there should also be suggestive historical evidence and support from attempts at its elimination from the patient's diet if appropriate.

The same comments apply to interpretation of the prick, scratch and intradermal tests, as these demonstrate bound IgE antibody on cutaneous mast cells. The results of these tests are obvious soon after doing them and they are cheap to do. However, they are not as sensitive as RAST tests and

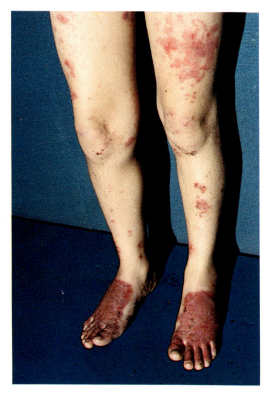

Figure 164 Allergic contact dermatitis caused by paraphenylenediamine in shoes in a child with atopic dermatitis.

not as easy to do in the child. It should be noted that a positive test to house dust is taken by some to be an important diagnostic feature of atopic dermatitis.

Evolution   Atopic dermatitis usually begins in the first year of life and often towards the end of the third or fourth month. Some cases start earlier but in these patients the diagnosis is usually made with hindsight because of the difficulty in differentiating seborrhoeic dermatitis. The absence of scratching, which starts at the end of the third month, also makes the differentiation difficult. If atopic dermatitis doesn't regress in the first year of life, as it does in very mild cases, it lasts on average some four or five years, but can last very much longer – even decades. It pursues a relapsing course with periods of worsening in spring and autumn and improvement during summer in the typical European climate. The periodic aggravation is itself inconsistent with varying degrees of severity of the rash. After an episode has subsided further relapses tend to be more brief, maybe only lasting a few weeks in the months of April and May.

Table 3

	Atopic dermatitis	Seborrhoeic dermatitis	Napkin dermatitis with secondary spread
Age of onset	Third month or later	First month	First month onwards
History of atopic disorder	In 70%	In 10%	In 10%
Pruritus	Yes	No, or mild	No, or mild
Initial sites	Face	Scalp and inguino-anal region	Inguino-anal region
Central facial localization	No	Yes	No
Flexural localization	Yes	Yes	No

More uncommonly the initial attack of atopic dermatitis starts at the age of three or four or even later. In general these patients have a low IgE level and do not have asthma as an associated complaint. These patients' atopic dermatitis tends to be persistent.

Very rarely atopic dermatitis starts in the second or third decade of life (Figures 165, 166). If a detailed history is taken from these patients it is often revealed that in fact they have suffered from brief episodes of dermatitis. These individuals may not only have the typical flexural lesions but also have lesions on the hands and superimposed contact dermatitis.

Prognosis For the most part, parents not only want to know that the disease will eventually clear, they want to know when. Of course it is not possible to be categoric but at least it is certain that if the disorder affects localized area only, such as the face, the outlook is much better than if the disease is generalized. It is also true that the disorder tends to persist for longer in children in whom the disease first appeared after the age of two. It appears that boys are predominantly affected in the first year of life and that girls predominate in cases that last for ten years or longer. The total IgE level has no significance for the prognosis, and as was pointed out previously a seriously affected patient may have low, normal or high IgE levels. Association with other atopic manifestations, especially asthma, and predisposition to infection, have more significance. These conditions are associated with elevation of the IgE levels and with a T-lymphocyte deficit.

Treatment Although atopic dermatitis is a disease in which hypersensitivities have some importance, the disorder cannot be counted as an 'allergic' disease in the classical sense. This is so because the disease cannot be removed by allergen avoidance, for example diet, or by desensitization procedures. However, some patients do seem to benefit to some degree by removal of one or the other dietary allergen – especially children with early onset disease, in whom cow's milk and eggs seem to play some aggravating role. As mentioned previously, these children can be identified from the history and trial elimination diets. The roles of house dust mites and pollen antigens is also unclear in patients who have positive skin or RAST tests. Certainly some workers have claimed that elimination of house dust mites from the bedrooms of affected children, whether by assiduous vacuum cleaning or by sprays of an anti-aspergillus (the foodstuff of the house dust mite) antibiotic (natamycin) greatly improves the eczematous condition.

Because of the ease with which the skin of patients with atopic dermatitis becomes infected and the functional deficit in T-suppressor lymphocytes, the disorder has been interpreted as a minimal immuno-deficiency syndrome and many attempts at treatment with immuno-stimulants have been made. However, in general, the results of trials of levamisole, transfer factor and thymopoietin pentapeptide (TP5) have not looked very promising. It is difficult to evaluate the isolated case in whom improvement has occurred after treatment, as the disease so frequently spontaneously fluctuates in intensity.

It should be emphasized that it is important to have a long chat with the parents before prescribing anything. They should know the course of the disease, the aggravating factors, and its complications. The parents must be reassured that their child will in fact improve and will not be scarred or disfigured. They should also be instructed in the practical issues of general care and specific treatments. Such advice and reassurance need to be reinforced at intervals while the child is being supervised by the clinic.

It must always be remembered that the disease has a protracted but relapsing course so that treatments should only be prescribed with due regard to the potentially harmful effects of long term administration. When the disease is severe or there are complications, systemic treatment

Figure 165 Atopic dermatitis in an adult with flexural involvement.

Figure 166 Atopic dermatitis in an adult with impetiginization of the folds.

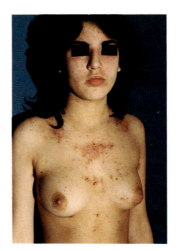

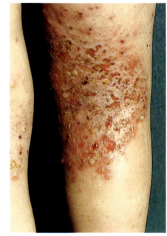

may be required. Systemic antibiotics are needed at the first sign of impetiginization and when the disease shows extensive exudation. Some believe that staphylococcus has a particular role in the aggravation of the disease and give erythromycin for six months of the year or benzathine penicillin by injection every seven to ten days. In rare patients with established hypogammaglobulinaemia, some benefit may accrue from administration of gammaglobulin at regular intervals.

Antihistamines are widely prescribed for atopic dermatitis. Their main use is their sedative action for hyperexcitable and itchy children who do not sleep, and don't allow their parents to sleep. In these patients one or other of the antihistamines should be given for a ten to fifteen day period, and it is worth changing the particular drug on subsequent occasions. Some of the newer antihistamines have less of a sedative effect and these may be less useful for atopic dermatitis patients because of this. H_2 blocking agents such as cimetidine and ranitidine seem to offer little help to this group of patients.

Figure 167 Atopic dermatitis in an adult.

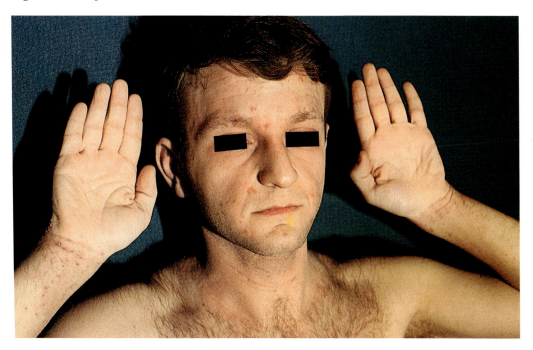

Disodium cromoglycate is not well absorbed when given by mouth and does not seem to help atopic dermatitis. One study claimed good effects from a topical preparation of 10 per cent sodium cromoglycate but this has not been confirmed.

Systemic corticosteroids are infrequently used because of the side effects, both short term (Figure 168) and long term, on growth, as these drugs have to be administered over long periods for this chronic disease. Although children can be kept symptom free with systemic corticosteroids, the cost in stunting of growth, striae, susceptibility to infection and adrenal insufficiency after unexpected stress or illness is unacceptable unless life is intolerable without them.

Topical corticosteroids may also cause unpleasant side effects, but they do give considerable relief and permit healing of the dermatitic skin with its disordered barrier. Clearly a balance must be struck between the relief from the distressing pruritus and the vulnerability of the damaged skin on the one hand and the potential hazards from the use of topical corticosteroids on the other.

To assist in the prescription of the topical corticosteroids the following guidelines are offered:

- They should not be used in the inguino-anal region, especially in the first two years of life, when plastic pants act as an occlusive dressing.
- Only bland unmedicated creams or hydrocortisone should be allowed on the face, in general, and around the eyes in particular.

- The preparation should only be used on the lesions and not on the surrounding skin.
- These preparations should not be used for itching alone, or on areas of transient erythema. They should be restricted to inflamed lesions that have been present for at least two days.
- The topical corticosteroids should not be used more frequently than twice per day and for not more than five consecutive days per week. It has been demonstrated that maximum saturation of the receptors occurs at this time and there is no further benefit if treatment is given continuously for longer.
- The dosage should be regulated by explaining to the parents how long a tube should last and how much (for example, of cream squeezed from the tube) should be used at each application.
- Warning should be given of the skin pallor due to vasoconstriction that occurs after use of the corticosteroids.

If these hints are built into a treatment regimen, serious side effects are unlikely and treatment with topical corticosteroids will give good results.

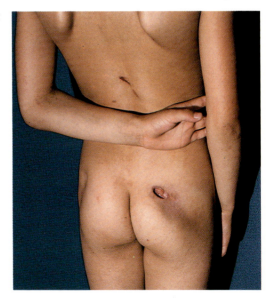

Figure 168 Atrophy and ulceration following injection of triamcinolone for atopic dermatitis.

Bland emollients without any active ingredient are also extremely useful – especially for areas of dry skin and hyperkeratosis. Tar preparations are particularly useful for areas of lichenification.

Prophylaxis Paediatricians advise continuing breast feeding as long as possible to inhibit the development of atopy in general and atopic dermatitis in particular. Strong evidence in support of this contention is in short supply and more rigorously controlled and prolonged studies are required. Any measure to decrease the itch is important. For example, clothes made of fine cotton and linen are less provoking to itch than coarse woolly-type materials. Similarly, circumstances that provoke sweating should be avoided. The skin of the atopic is generally dry and rough or scaly, and this tendency should not be aggravated by frequent hot baths. For the same reason, emollient cleansing agents should be used instead of ordinary soap.

As mentioned previously, the barrier function of the skin of atopic dermatitis patients is disturbed and there are decreased immune defences. For these reasons patients should avoid contact with individuals who have any form of skin infection – and in particular herpes simplex. It is also wise to avoid contact with applications containing strong sensitizers such as neomycin, antihistamines and sulphonamides. They should also avoid contact with irritant substances such as soaps and detergents, as these may also aggravate the condition. Such children should not plan to enter occupations in which the skin is constantly exposed to chemical and mechanical trauma, such as catering, hairdressing, building and mechanical engineering.

Another aspect of prophylaxis concerns the development of asthma. Some 25 per cent of children with atopic dermatitis develop asthma. It appears that asthma is more common, when the dermatitis starts very early in life, in children who exprience recurrent chest infections, whose parents are heavy smokers, and who have raised IgE levels. Avoidance of carpets and curtains in their bedrooms, and of woollen bed clothes, furry toys and domestic animals may also be helpful.

Allergic contact dermatitis

The frequency of occurence of this disorder is exactly the reverse of atopic dermatitis. It is quite exceptional to see the disease in the first three years, but it becomes more frequent with increasing years. Contact allergy appears after a variable number of contacts with a sensitizer. The rash appears at the site of contact but may spread to involve other areas. Among the most common sensitizers are the paraphenlyenediamines. These are dyes often found in shoes, and are responsible for allergic contact dermatitis of the feet (Figure 169). Chrome salts, nickel and topical medicaments, amongst which the most frequent are sulphonamides (Figure 170), antihistamines and neomycin, may also cause the reaction.

Treatment   This is directed to detection of the allergen by patch testing and advice as to its avoidance. Local treatment is similar to that for the other eczematous disorders (for example, atopic dermatitis).

Figure 169 Allergic contact dermatitis of the feet due to dyes in shoes.

Figure 170 Allergic contact dermatitis caused by a sulphonamide.

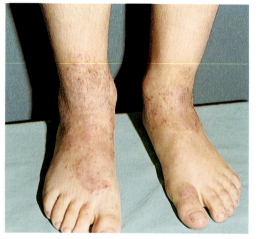
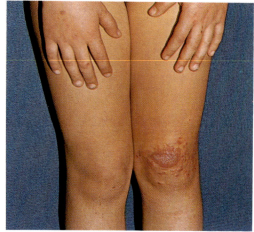

Pityriasis alba (pityriasis simplex)

This disorder of uncertain nature is common in children of school age. The lesions are paler than the surrounding skin (Figure 171) but may start off being pink in colour. The affected areas are covered in a fine pityriasiform scale. Lesions are mostly found on the face, but may occur on the upper arms and elsewhere on the limbs. The disorder often starts at the end of the summer season but this may only be because of the contrast of the affected area with surrounding tanned skin. It becomes less apparent with the loss of suntan, to recur in the following year. Some individuals seem to depigment very easily after minor traumata and this may partially explain the odd appearance of these lesions. The disorder is very resistant to treatment but usually clears after some months without specific therapy.

Figure 171 Pityriasis alba in a child of seven.

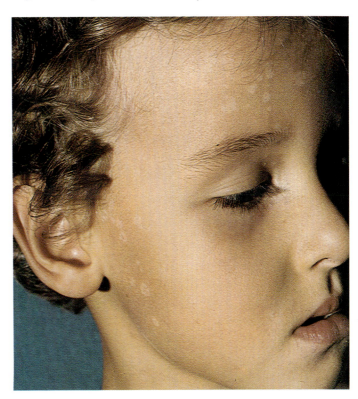

Geographic tongue

This quite common disorder seems to occur more frequently in atopics. The initial lesion is a whitish area that rapidly enlarges by extending peripherally assuming bizarre figurate patterns (Figure 172). Lesions tend to recur frequently in the first year of life, the frequency of recurrence lessening with the passing of years. It may 'flare' during pyrexial illness, especially with upper respiratory tract infections.

Geographic tongue is generally asymptomatic and no treatment is required apart from that needed to reassure the parents. The significance and pathogenesis of this odd disorder are unknown, although some consider it a lingual equivalent of pityriasis alba or an eczematide.

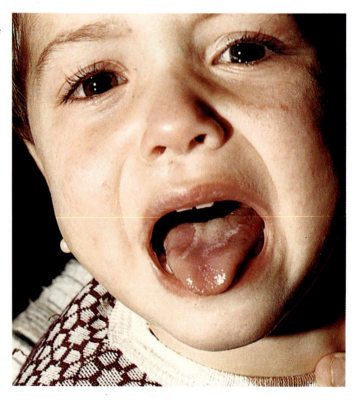

Figure 172 Geographic tongue. Note the configuration of the lesions.

Geographic tongue has to be distinguished from other recurrent lesions that affect the buccal mucosa, including aphthous ulceration and fixed drug eruption. Aphthae of the buccal cavity are also of uncertain nature and tend to be familial. Aphthae may be single or multiple, each having a diameter of 3 to 5 mm (Figure 173) although larger lesions 2 to 3 cm in diameter are occasionally seen. They have a sloughy, yellowish floor and are surrounded by an erythematous halo. Each lesion lasts seven to ten days. Recurrences can happen as frequently as every ten to fifteen days. They are easily distinguished from other lesions because of the discomfort they cause and their sensitivity to spicy foods.

Figure 173 Typical aphthae of tongue, showing a depressed, yellowish base and an erythematous halo.

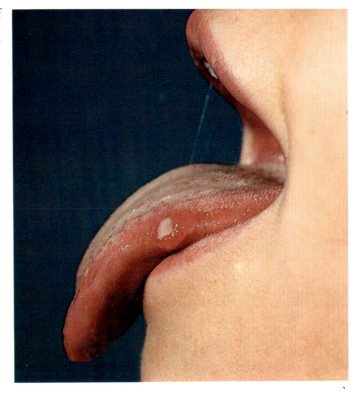

Fixed drug eruption of the buccal cavity (see page 128) provokes intense discomfort, making eating difficult. Clinically, large areas of macerated and eroded mucosae are found in this condition. Fixed drug eruption frequently involves the lips, leaving a violet or lead discoloration. Non-recurrent disorders that affect the mouth, such as herpes simplex or herpangina, are in general easier to distinguish from geographic tongue.

Urticaria

The typical lesion is the weal – a raised, whitish or pink lesion (Figure 175). Weals are usually well defined and surrounded by erythema. The important distinguishing feature is that the weal is transient, lasting only a few hours and disappearing without trace. This is not always the case in children, in whom there may be some residual pigmentation due to the outpouring of a bloody exudate in severe cases.

Intense itching usually accompanies urticaria – in very young children the itching may be mild even when there is severe urticaria. Persistent urticaria lasting months or years is less frequent in young children. Acute urticaria, lasting a few hours only, is more common in atopics and is the result of allergic hypersensitivity being mediated by IgE.

The foods that most frequently cause urticaria in the first years of life are peaches, fish, milk, eggs, walnuts and hazel nuts. It is common for these patients to have angioedema of the eyes and lips (Figure 176). The tissues

Figure 174 Acute urticaria in a child of six. Note the presence of purpura.

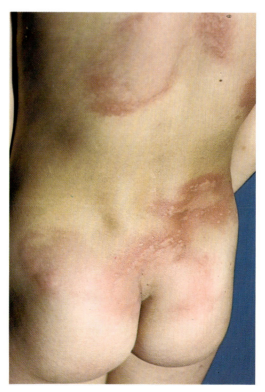

of these sites are particularly lax and are prone to swellings caused by oedema of the skin.

This type of allergic angioedema must be differentiated from the angioedema due to C^1 esterase inhibitor deficiency. This condition is much more severe, may be accompanied by intestinal colic, and can in fact be fatal.

Urticaria in children may also accompany a febrile episode of upper respiratory tract infection. In these cases the urticaria may be due to the lowering of the threshold to urticarial lesions by the pyrexia or due to administration of salicylates which provoke the release of histamines.

Chronic urticaria may last months or years, and in these patients it is extremely difficult to find the underlying cause. Clinical examination and laboratory studies do not usually assist in detecting any underlying abnormality. It is important, however, to exclude rare causes of urticaria such as that seen in immune complex nephropathy. Gastrointestinal parasites are sometimes responsible for the disorder, although they account for a very small proportion of the total number of patients. The physical urticarias, including urticaria due to heat or pressure and dermographic urticaria, are rare causes below the age of one year.

Treatment   Clearly the best course of action is to remove the underlying cause if it is known. For example, when urticaria is due to a food

Figure 175 Urticarial weal. Note the prominence of the weals.

Figure 176 Allergic angioedema of the eyelids in an atopic subject.

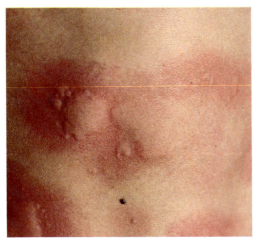
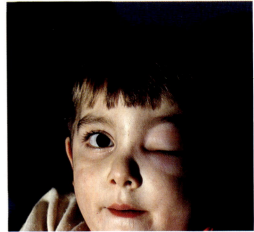

126

hypersensitivity, the responsible allergen should be removed from the diet or particular preparative procedures avoided.

Symptomatic measures are needed at times. Antihistamines are helpful if there are many and frequent lesions. Steroids and even subcutaneous adrenaline (epinephrine) may be required as life saving measures for anaphylactic shock and angioedema with glottal involvement. Oral steroids should not be given for chronic idiopathic urticaria – the antihistamines are sufficient if treatment is required.

In a proportion of patients it is worth trying to eliminate drugs and foodstuffs containing colorants and preservatives that cause liberation of histamine — salicylates, tartrazine (FD & C Yellow No 5) and benzoates.

In children affected by hereditary angioedema (C^1 esterase inhibitor deficiency) the administration of synthetic androgens and epsilon amino caproic acid prevents attacks. The acute attacks can be treated by infusion of purified inhibitors of C^1 esterase.

Fixed drug eruption

Practitioners and paediatricians rarely recognize this entity (Figures 179, 180) despite the usual ease with which this condition can be identified. After taking a drug (or occasionally a constituent of food) that previously did not cause any side effect, one or two intensely erythematous patches occur on the skin and on the anogenital mucosae. If the provocative drug is identified or stopped, the affected area becomes less red in a few days and the patches develop a brownish pigmentation that may persist for as long as some months. If the drug responsible is given again after a period that may vary from half an hour to twenty-four hours (in mild cases) the previously affected sites become inflamed again and even bullae can occur.

Figures 177 and 178 Fixed drug eruption on thigh before (Figure 177) and during (Figure 178) a challenge test with sulphamethoxypyridazine, demonstrating the reddening of the pre-existing area.

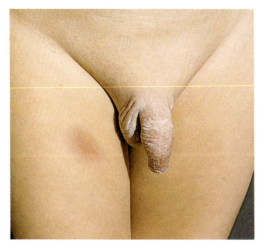 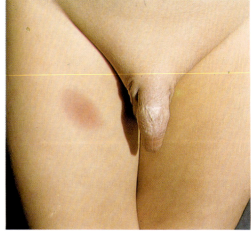

It is sometimes difficult for the patient to identify the responsible drug as it is often an analgesic, antipyretic or laxative preparation that he or she has taken for many years and which is thought to be innocent. In children under the age of ten, sulphonamides and pyrazolidine type drugs are often the cause. A common mistake is to believe that the child is allergic to several drugs because the reaction occurs after several preparations. However, in these cases it is frequently the inclusion of the same drug in several different preparations that is responsible. It is important to identify the offending drug and for this reason it is wise to admit the child for 'challenge tests' in which the suspected drugs are given sequentially, so that the particular drug can be identified and subsequently avoided.

Figure 179 and 180 Fixed drug eruption due to pyramidone in a child of eleven. The eruption was not recognized and the child underwent a sternal puncture and a muscle biopsy as a blood dyscrasia was suspected.

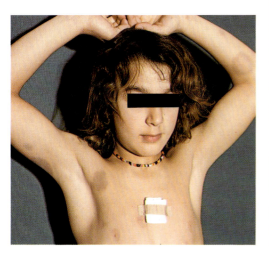

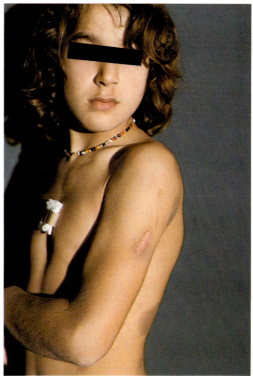

Anaphylactoid purpura (Henoch-Schönlein purpura)

This disorder is a vasculitis which affects the skin, joints, intestine and kidneys. The skin lesions are important in reaching the correct diagnosis. Typically they are polymorphic with purpuric, erythematous and papular elements (Figure 181). Figurate lesions are quite often seen (Figure 183), but nodular lesions (Figure 181) are uncommon. Lesions with superficial necrosis are also quite unusual (Figure 184). As with most of the vasculitic disorders, the skin lesions are most in evidence over the legs, presumably because of postural considerations.

An attack characteristically lasts some ten to twenty days and further attacks occur at intervals of from three to twelve months. In some cases – often those which are precipitated by an upper respiratory tract infection – the attacks are separated by longer intervals or do not recur.

Figure 181 Anaphylactoid purpura. Small lesions of the legs.

Figure 182 Anaphylactoid purpura with ecchymotic nodules.

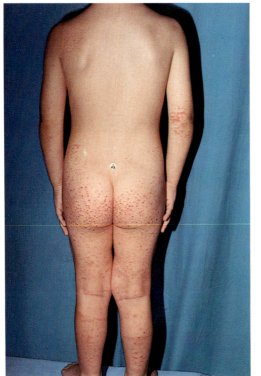

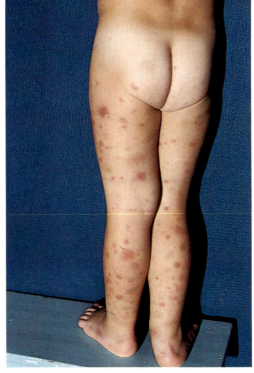

130

The disease is rare below the age of two and mostly affects children and adolescents.

Aetiopathogenesis   The vasculitis seems to be the result of IgA immune complexes but the aetiology of these is obscure. Although a streptococcal infection may be suspected it is rare to confirm this clinically or by laboratory tests.

Treatment   There are no effective treatments, so that rest in bed remains the best remedy. Antihistamines may give some slight relief. Corticosteroid treatment is only indicated in severe disease with involvement of other organs.

Figure 183 Anaphylactoid purpura with figurate target shaped lesions in a young infant.

Figure 184 Superficial necrotic lesions due to anaphylactoid purpura in a boy aged twelve.

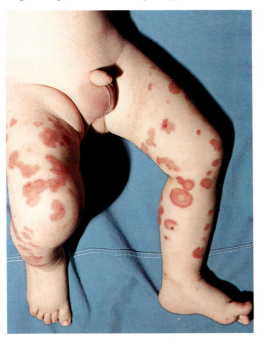

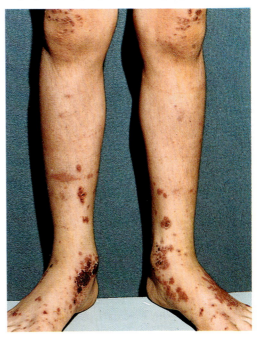

Seborrhoeic dermatitis

Seborrhoeic dermatitis is seen most frequently in the first three months of life. While it is usually a trivial disease, far more severe varieties do occur, which may even be life threatening.

The name derives from the distribution of lesions, which is similar to the same disease in the adult, that is, the scalp, the glabella and medial margins of the eyebrow, the central facial region and the retroauricular region. However, some sites of involvement in the adult – the sternal and interscapular regions – are never involved in children. The inguino-anal region is also affected in children, probably because of the trauma that this area sustains from the use of napkins. The appearance of the scalp lesions (Figure 185) with whitish-yellow scaling also resembles that seen in adults and further validates the use of the term.

There is no evidence to link a seborrhoeic constitution in the parents with the development of seborrhoeic dermatitis in the child. Neither is there any evidence that children with seborrhoeic dermatitis develop any seborrhoeic complaints as adults. It should be noted that the sebaceous glands of neonates are functional due to androgenic stimulation from maternal hormones. There is no relation to the hormonal problems that occur in the neonate (Figure 186). The seborrhoeic glands become quiescent after three months of life.

Figure 185 Seborrhoeic dermatitis. Typical scaling lesions over the scalp, with yellowish scale affecting the glabella and the medial thirds of the eyebrows.

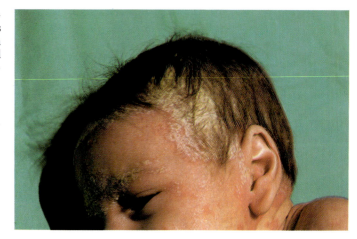

Symptoms The sexes are equally affected and the disorder may be seen as early as the second week of life. In mildly affected cases there may only be a few scaling crusted areas in the scalp ('milk crusts'). In more severe cases other areas are involved as indicated above. Commonly, erythematous and exudative lesions coexist in the inguino-anal region but areas behind the ears, on the neck and in the axillae are usually first to be involved. Sometimes, and as in napkin dermatitis, secondary psoriasiform lesions appear on the trunk and limbs (Figure 187). These lesions may become confluent and affect much of the skin surface.

It is not certain whether the condition known eponymously as Leiner's disease should be included in a general description of seborrhoeic dermatitis or not. This is a generalized inflammatory dermatosis occurring in neonates of less than three months which can be extremely serious. In the earliest stages of this disorder (Figure 188), very inflamed lesions of the face and of the inguino-anal region are seen. These are followed by a punctate eruption of the trunk and limbs. In a few days the punctate

Figure 186 Pustules on the face of a neonate ascribed to hormonal alterations occurring at this time.

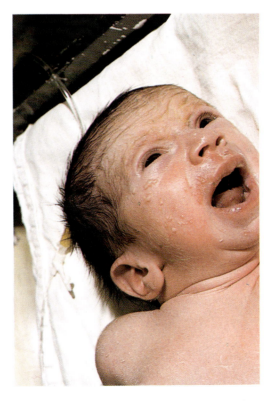

lesions enlarge and coalesce, giving rise to the erythrodermic picture (Figure 189) that persists for some seven to fifteen days, to resolve with scaling without recurring.

Natural History   Seborrhoeic dermatitis usually regresses before the age of five months and some authorities doubt whether the entity can occur after this age.

Differential diagnosis   For the differential diagnosis from atopic dermatitis and napkin dermatitis see page 112. Histiocytosis X can involve the 'seborrhoeic sites' but the lesions are papular and often haemorrhagic. Any desquamative dermatitis of the scalp may be difficult to distinguish but when due to other causes usually begins after the age of five months.

Figure 187 Psoriasiform seborrhoeic dermatitis.

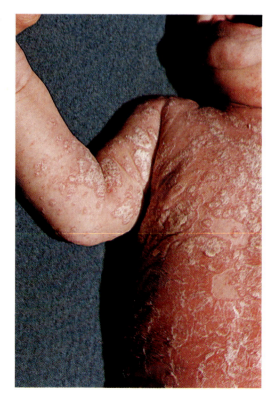

Other causes of scaling scalp usually affect the central part of the scalp region and occasionally the face.

At other times there may be multiple well-delineated, psoriasiform, isolated scaling spots or confluent areas which may persist unchanged for several years, improving in the summer and deteriorating in the winter. The similarity of these various disorders to seborrhoeic dermatitis depends on the distribution of the eruption. Atopic dermatitis is one disorder that gives rise to such lesions and in the first few months can mimic seborrhoeic dermatitis of the scalp. Similarly children aged two to ten with typical atopic dermatitis or other atopic disorder can develop an itching scaly rash of the scalp.

Another group of disorders that may cause scaling in the scalp region are the ichthyotic disorders. Autosomal dominant or sex linked ichthyosis can

Figure 188 Inflamed dermatitis of the face and inguino-anal region in which there are punctate lesions.

Figure 189 The same boy as in figure 188 two days later. Confluent erythematous lesions of the trunk and limbs (Leiner's disease).

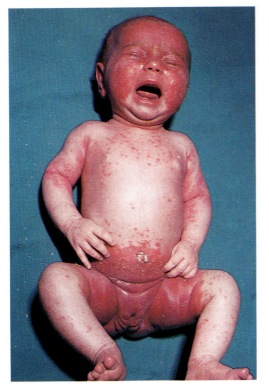

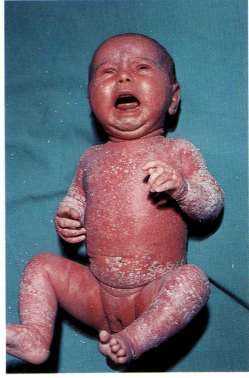

be distinguished by the generalized roughening of the skin surface with accentuation over the lower legs, where there may be larger, darker adherent scales.

Psoriasis can also begin with isolated multiple scalp lesions, although these are usually small and rounded. Sometimes all of these disorders can be excluded, and in a prepubertal child it is probably better not to make a firm diagnosis rather than attaching the label seborrhoeic dermatitis if there are no corroborating features.

Treatment In mildly affected patients, removal of scales with oil is sufficient. When the flexures are affected, non-irritant antimicrobial agents should be used (for example povidone-iodine preparations) to clean the affected areas, followed by an emollient, calamine cream or, if necessary, a weak corticosteroid. Following removal of the scale a hydrocortisone preparation should be applied with due regard to the

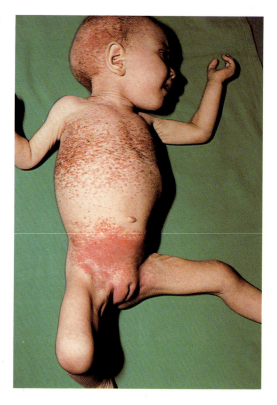

Figure 190 Histiocytosis X (Letterer-Siwe disease). Haemorrhagic micropapular lesions confluent in the inguinal and scalp regions resembling seborrhoeic dermatitis.

hazards of treatment with topical corticosteroids (see treatment of atopic dermatitis). In Leiner's disease, care should be taken that the erythroderma is not responsible for a serious loss of heat. Attention should also be paid to other possibly systemic effects.

Psoriasis

This disease affects some 2 per cent of the population but is less frequent in the early years of life.

Aetiology Hereditary factors seem to be important (Figure 191) although the exact mode of inheritance is uncertain.

Clinical features The lesions are reddened, of variable size and covered by thick white scale that seems to become whiter if the lesions are scratched (Figures 193–196). The sites affected include the extensor

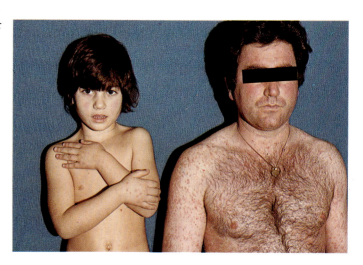

Figure 191 Psoriasis in father and son.

aspects of the elbows and knees and the scalp. In children psoriasis is often eruptive with small lesions.

It is not clear whether napkin psoriasis should be included in this chapter or not. After some weeks from the start of ordinary napkin dermatitis – usually at the fourth or fifth month of life – secondary, more scaly lesions appear over the trunk and limbs. The lesions, which are punctate, at first enlarge peripherally until the rash becomes confluent, involving much of the skin surface (Figure 192). This odd, psoriasiform rash usually clears after four to five weeks and does not recur even though the napkin dermatitis may return. Some authorities believe that the disease represents a type of premature psoriasis in an individual with a psoriatic diathesis and who has a napkin dermatitis, but there is no strong evidence for this view.

Evolution   In the majority of sufferers from psoriasis the disease is life-long. It tends to improve in the summer and worsens in the winter. It should be remembered that in about one fifth of children who have eruptive psoriasis the disorder can regress, not to recur subsequently.

Pustular psoriasis in children (Figure 197) is a serious complication of the disorder in which the skin is covered by large numbers of sterile micro-pustules.

Treatment   It must be remembered that the disorder persists and treatments may have to be continued for long periods. Reassurance of the parents and the young patient to the effect that psoriasis is not contagious

Figure 192 Extensive psoriasiform napkin dermatitis.

Figure 193 Psoriasis. Typical psoriasis with heaped up scaling.

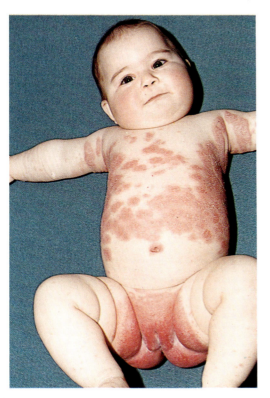

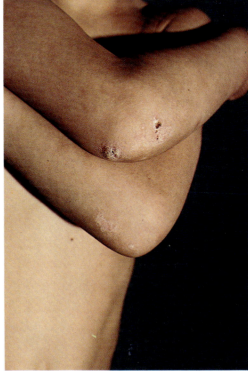

and is compatible with excellent general health is both important and helpful in management.

The problem for the majority of sufferers from psoriasis is an aesthetic one and the parents should be reminded that their attitudes, and those of all who come into close contact with the child, will influence his or her own self-esteem and confidence. The young patient should be encouraged not to be obsessed by the disease but if possible to accept and live in harmony with the disability – which after all, for the majority of patients, is not a serious problem.

In the treatment of psoriasis the physician has to bear in mind that each

Figure 194 Typical scaling red lesions of psoriasis of the legs.

Figure 195 Psoriasis in a child of fourteen months who doesn't seem unduly troubled by his disorder.

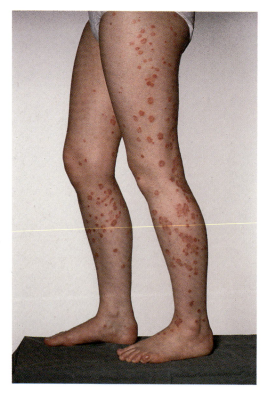

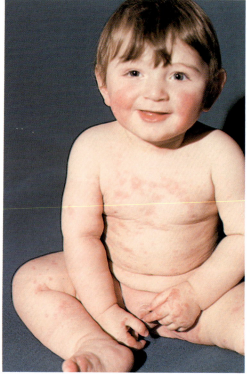

patient may respond differently. However, one treatment that seems to aid most sufferers is exposure to sunlight. Mildly affected patients may only need to be involved in some outdoor sport to have sufficient sun exposure to remain clear of lesions. This should be carefully explained to the child as the natural tendency is to 'cover up' as much as possible to hide the blemishes.

In general, photochemotherapy using long wave ultraviolet irradiation (UVA) and photosensitizing psoralens (so-called PUVA) is contraindicated in children because of the potentially harmful long-term side effects. Systemic corticosteroids are also strongly contraindicated. They may

Figure 196 Psoriasis in a child of seven years.

Figure 197 Pustular psoriasis.

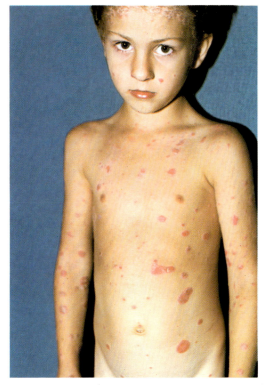

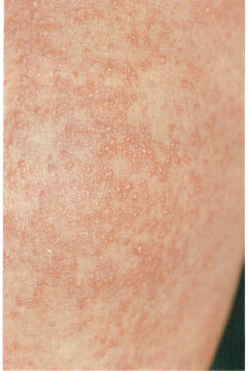

produce temporary benefit but at a cost of unpleasant and potentially hazardous side effects. The same considerations apply to the use of potent topical corticosteroids. If these latter preparations are to be used at all in psoriasis their use should be restricted to certain areas (exposed areas) and for extremely short periods (see treatment of atopic dermatitis).

A useful approach is first to remove the scale on the lesions with 2–6 per cent salicylic acid in white soft paraffin (petrolatum) and then to treat with tar preparations (2–6 per cent) or dithranol (anthralin) preparations (0.1–2 per cent).

Alopecia areata

This is one of the commonest dermatological disorders of children. Its importance is in its chronicity, its lack of response to treatment and the cosmetic problems that it causes.

Aetiology Some clinicians believe that psychosomatic factors are important and point to the increased incidence of nocturnal enuresis in affected children and the presence of psychological disorders in this group of patients. However, it is clear that other factors are concerned as there is an undoubted familial predisposition to the disease and associations with organ specific autoimmune diseases.

Signs and symptoms Rounded hairless patches some 2 to 10 cm in diameter are characteristic of the disease (Figures 198, 199). The hairless skin appears normal as do the follicular mouths. The hairs at the periphery of the affected patches are easily distracted and leave a stump of hair that has a characteristic exclamation-mark-like profile. The loss of hair may extend to the eyebrows and eyelashes.

Natural history It is difficult to know whether any treatment is effective, as spontaneous remission is common. Regrowth of hair is much

Figure 198 Alopecia areata showing affected area 3–4 cm in diameter. Note the absence of erythema or other abnormality.

Figure 199 Alopecia areata. The normal hair has been cut short in this patient.

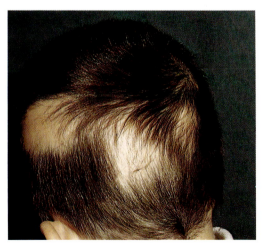

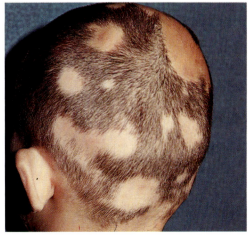

Figure 200 Three year old child before the disorder.

Figure 201 The same child six months later with alopecia totalis.

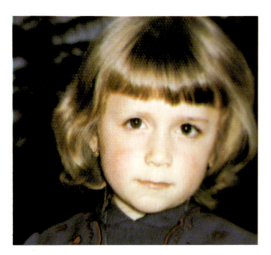

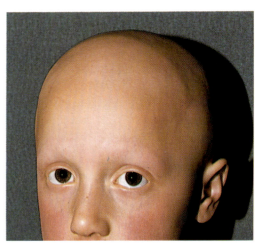

Figure 202 The same child aged four, some two months after starting systemic corticosteroid treament.

Figure 203 The same child, now aged four and a half years. When the corticosteroid treatment was stopped the alopecia recurred and treatment with atopical corticosteroids was started.

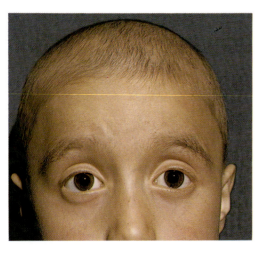

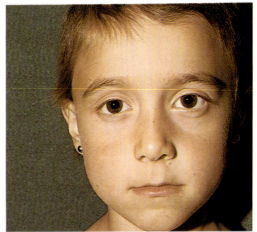

more common when there are only a few small patches. When the disease is very extensive regrowth tends to be less complete and recurrence more frequent. In these patients the disease may last for years. When the disease involves the nape of the neck and the periphery of the scalp (ophiasiform alopecia) the outlook is poor and total loss of hair follows frequently (alopecia totalis) (Figures 201, 204).

Differential diagnosis In tinea capitis the hairs tend to break off some 3 to 4 mm from the scalp surface and there are signs of inflammation of the skin. In trichotillomania and in alopecia due to trauma the affected area is not usually rounded and there are broken hairs of different lengths. Aplasia cutis is a congenital disorder in which the hairless skin is thin, depressed and atrophic.

Treatment Treatment is inadvisable for a few localized areas of alopecia and the significance of the disorder should be played down by the physician. When the disorder is slightly more extensive topical cortico-steroids may be used but are rarely successful. If topical corticosteroids are used, the same rules apply as for atopic dermatitis (see page 98). Atrophy of the scalp skin is often seen after the use of potent topical corticosteroids for this condition (Figure 205) but is reversible.

Treatment with sensitization by DNCB or some other sensitizing agent had a vogue, but is uncomfortable, inconvenient and only partially and temporarily helpful. Local treatment of any kind is hardly ever helpful

Figure 204 Alopecia univer-salis.

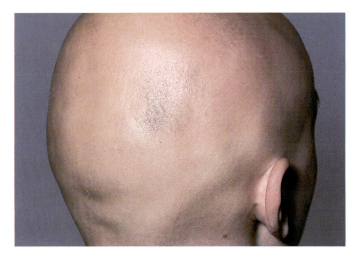

145

when there is 50 per cent hair loss or more. Systemic steroids in a dose of 0.5 mg prednisone per kg body weight per day for one month, with reduction subsequently, is sometimes helpful but relapse is frequent. If the disorder can be controlled by a small dose (for example, prednisone 5 mg daily) it may be worth persisting with the treatment, weighing up the potentially dangerous side effects against the undoubted psychological benefits.

For some cases the best and indeed the only treatment is with a wig.

Figure 205 Skin atrophy from the use of a topical cortico-steroid for the treatment of alopecia areata. The skin is thinned and dermal blood vessels show through it.

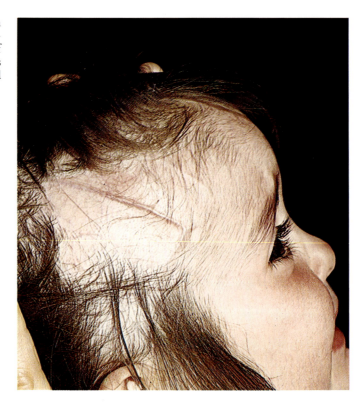

Vitiligo

This common disorder is characterized by the presence of white areas on the skin surface caused by the loss of melanin in the affected area. A systematized form exists (Figure 206) in which white spots occur symmetrically on the hands, eyebrows, perigenital region and other areas. A nerve root distribution can also be observed (Figure 207).

Cause   The cause is unknown but familial and neural factors are probably involved. Recently evidence has come to light suggesting that auto-

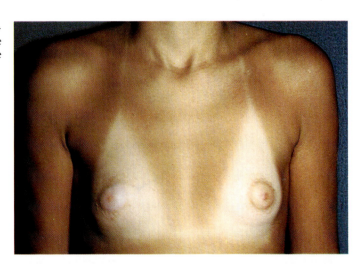

Figure 206 Systematized vitiligo in a child of twelve. Note the depigmentation of the nipple.

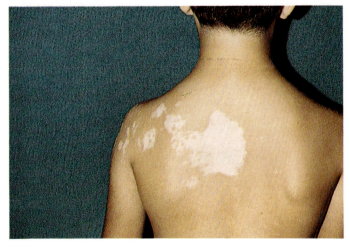

Figure 207 Vitiligo in a neural distribution involving the left scapula and deltoid region.

immune factors are involved. Vitiligo is associated with autoimmune diseases, including hyperthyroidism and diabetes; even in the absence of overt autoimmune disease there is an increased prevalence of auto-antibodies.

Natural history In the systematized variety the depigmented areas gradually spread so that all pigmentation gradually disappears. However the neural form tends to persist unchanged at the same sites.

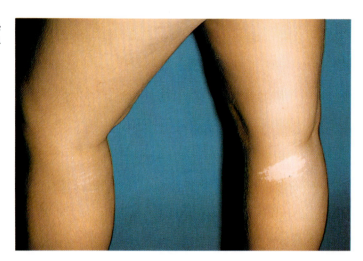

Figure 208 Vitiligo at the site of an elasticated band in a sock.

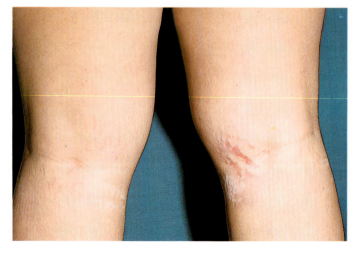

Figure 209 Local steroid treatment has improved the vitiligo but has caused unpleasant livid striae.

Treatment   The disorder is obvious and disfiguring so that it is frequent for patients to press hard for some kind of treatment.

For patients with widespread vitiligo photochemotherapy can be tried. Psoralens are given two hours before exposure to sunlight. The psoralens are usually given by mouth but topical preparations have also been used. In successfully treated patients the pigmentation begins at the follicles and spreads outwards and persists even after treatment has stopped. Unfortunately not all patients respond in this way. Some do not repigment at all, and others do so only transitorily. Care must be taken at the start of this treatment to avoid any overexposure and burning. Patients who do not respond to phototherapy should be warned not to have too much sun exposure as apart from the non-pigmented skin burning, the difference between the non-pigmented and the normally pigmented areas is accentuated.

For the more limited varieties of vitiligo topical corticosteroids can be tried with the same care to avoid side effects as mentioned previously under atopic dermatitis (see page 118) (Figures 208, 209).

Bullous dermatoses

Various autoimmune disorders are included under this general title. In these diseases it is believed that components of the dermo-epidermal junction or the epidermis stimulate the production of antibodies which later cause a bullous disorder at the same site. The pathogenetic significance of these autoantibodies is made plain by those cases of neonatal pemphigus in which the antibody and the disease are passed from mother to child. Pemphigus is an uncommon disease in which circulating antibodies to the intercellular epidermal zone can be detected in the blood of affected patients. The same is true for herpes gestationis – a rare bullous disorder seen in the last trimester of pregnancy. As might be expected from the transplacental passive transfer of antibodies the bullous disorder in the affected infant is transient and clears within a few weeks.

The most frequent vesiculo-bullous disorder of childhood is dermatitis

Figure 210 Herpes gestationis in a young woman and her son. The disorder was caused by the passive transfer of antibodies.

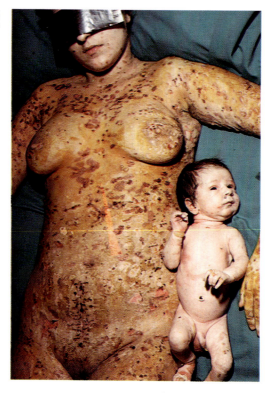

herpetiformis characterized by erythematous papular and urticated figurate lesions which are often rounded, annular or polycyclic and start a few millimetres in diameter but enlarge over a few days (Figure 211), with vesicles and bullae arising on these lesions in some instances. Application of iodine-containing preparations precipitates the appearance of bullae and can be used to help confirm the diagnosis. The lesions mostly occur on the trunk, around the axillae, on the knees and elbows and on the buttocks.

The disorder starts in early childhood (four to six years of age), is extremely chronic and lasts many years. Like adult dermatitis herpetiformis, it seems to have a strong association with gluten enteropathy. Some children with dermatitis herpetiformis present with symptoms due to malabsorption – about one third present with malabsorption syndrome

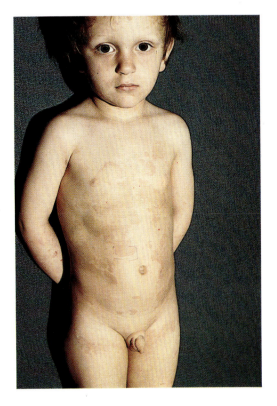

Figure 211 Figurate lesions and papules of dermatitis herpetiformis in a child of four years.

in the first year of life. In many children with dermatitis herpetiformis objective signs of malabsorption are not obvious but the disorder can be detected by laboratory tests and in particular jejunal biopsy.

The association of the skin and gut disorder may be explained by the finding of antibodies which cross react with a component of gluten (gliadin) and reticulin of skin and gut.

Treatment A gluten free diet seems to be useful in controlling both the gut and skin disorder but may take many months before being effective. Even though gastrointestinal symptoms are not clinically evident it is worthwhile instituting a gluten free diet. The drug diaminodiphenyl-sulphone (dapsone) in a dose of 1–2 mg per kg per day controls the skin manifestations in a dramatic way and is so efficacious within twenty-four to forty-eight hours that it has been used as a diagnostic test. Unfortunately, side effects are frequent as the drug causes methaemo-globinaemia, sulphaemoglobinaemia and haemolysis. The undesirable side effects are much more severe in individuals who are deficient in glucose 6 phosphate dehydrogenase and may make treatment with this drug impossible.

Rarer bullous disorders in childhood include pemphigoid (Figure 212), a chronic bullous disorder in which large bullae tend to occur on the entire skin surface, and chronic bullous disease in childhood, in which bullous lesions appear perigenitally.

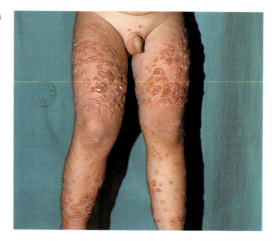

Figure 212 Pemphigoid in a child of two with large bullae on the lower limbs.

Connective tissue disorders (auto-immune diseases)

In the first twelve years of life connective tissue disorders are quite uncommon. The most prevalent of this group of diseases in childhood is scleroderma, which has to be distinguished from neonatal sclerema and scleroedema. A distinctive form of dermatomyositis occurs in childhood but lupus erythematosus, especially when confined to the skin, is rare. It should be noted that granuloma annulare is quite common in childhood and that the nodular form of the disorder can be confused with the nodules of rheumatoid arthritis.

Systemic lupus erythematosus (Figure 213) is sometimes observed in the second decade and may present with skin lesions to the dermatologist. The prognosis of this disorder has been much improved by the introduction of modern treatments including the use of corticosteroids and immunosuppressive drugs.

It is rare to see chronic discoid lupus erythematosus in childhood (Figure 214) as it is seen mostly in the third and fourth decades. It occurs in

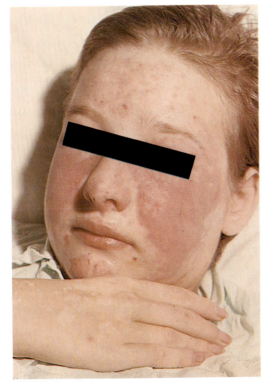

Figure 213 Systemic lupus erythematosus in a girl aged fourteen.

Figure 214 Discoid lupus erythematosus showing several fixed, reddened, hyperkeratotic lesions in a nine year old boy.

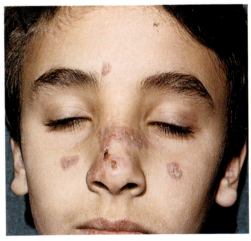

light exposed sites – mainly the face. The lesions are red, hyperkeratotic and atrophic and remain fixed for long periods. It is important that patients with the disorder avoid the sun, as sunlight aggravates the condition. Synthetic antimalarials or hydroxychloroquine, especially chloroquine, are often used in treatment.

Dermatomyositis in childhood differs from that in adults in several aspects. Children with the disease are much more likely to suffer from a systematized vasculitis and often have gastrointestinal complications that result from this. In children, dermatomyositis does not appear associated with any underlying neoplastic disorder, whereas in adults this is the case in approximately one fifth of patients.

Characteristically lilac red (heliotrope-coloured) patches appear on the face and round the eyes in particular. Similar areas appear on the limbs and on the backs of the fingers. Generally patients feel unwell and weak, and complain of pain and tenderness in the muscles of the limb girdles.

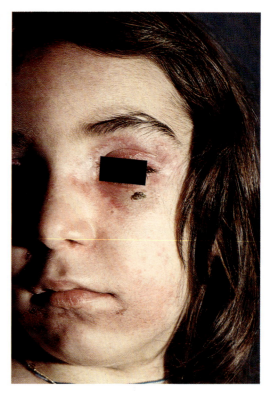

Figure 215 Dermatomyositis in a child of nine years. Note the characteristic lilac-pink colour of the eyebrows and eyelids.

Diagnosis may be established by the finding of elevated levels of muscle enzymes in the blood (aldolase or phosphocreatine kinase), an abnormal electromyogram or abnormal findings on muscle biopsy. The disorder does not respond well to treatment but some improvement may occur with systemic corticosteroids. Muscle contractures may occur as a sequel of the inflammation in muscle.

Scleroderma is the most common connective tissue disease of childhood – especially the skin manifestations. Usually the disease is localized (morphoea) but very rarely generalized forms are seen. The disease mostly occurs in isolated patches but linear and band-like forms are also seen. The affected skin is whitish, sclerotic, thickened and sometimes surrounded by an erythematous halo. Sometimes depressed atrophic lesions are found in which thinning of the skin occurs (Figure 217).

Linear lesions of morphoea do not respond well to treatment and the

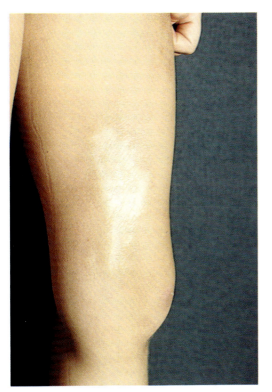

Figure 216 Scleroderma in a band-like distribution on the thigh. Note the white pearl-like appearance of the skin.

Figure 217 Band-like atrophy of the buttock.

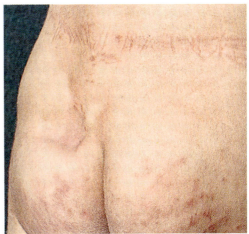

lesions may persist for long periods. Linear lesions tend to be particularly troublesome and may progress in extent for periods of a year or more. Otherwise morphoea may regress spontaneously within a period of a few years.

Rheumatoid nodules are sometimes seen in children with rheumatoid arthritis (Figure 218). They usually regress spontaneously or may be treated by intralesional injection of corticosteroids. These lesions are very difficult to distinguish histologically from the larger lesions of granuloma annulare which usually presents as small pink plaques or annuli. Lesions of granuloma annulare usually appear on the limbs (Figure 219) and last some weeks or months before spontaneously disappearing. Biopsy sometimes seems to provoke the disappearance of the lesion.

The cause is unknown but some authors have suggested that the disorder represents a hypersensitivity to bacterial antigens. In some cases there appears to be an association with diabetes, although the lesions that are seen when the association exists are special in that they are superficial and larger than usual.

Treatment Mostly this is not required, but topical corticosteroids and tar induce resolution in some cases if treatment is needed.

Figure 218 Rheumatoid nodule of thumb in child of five who did not have any arthritis.

Figure 219 Granuloma annulare of the wrist in a child aged four. There is a figurate lesion with a raised periphery.

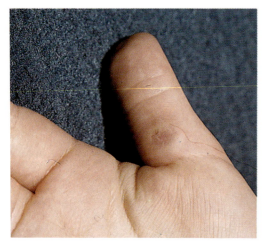

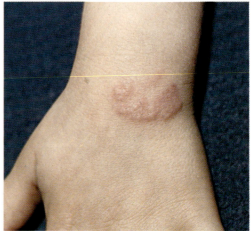

Mastocytosis (urticaria pigmentosa)

Cutaneous mastocytosis is characteristically a disease of children although more serious forms are occasionally seen in adults. Histologically lesions contain many mast cells. The latter are important cells in the inflammatory process and secrete histamine. This function explains the observation that the lesions spontaneously become urticated or require mild trauma before this happens (Figure 221). This sign gives rise to the term urticaria pigmentosa.

Cutaneous mastocytosis often presents at the age of six months with the appearance of brownish macules (macular mastocytosis) (Figure 223) or with brownish papules (papular mastocytosis) (Figure 224). More uncommonly isolated lesions occur (mast cell naevus). Rubbing the lesion induces an urticarial weal at the same site (Figure 221). If the induced inflammation is intense a blister may appear (Figure 222).

In the early years of life the sudden release of histamine into the circulation may cause reddening of the face (Figure 224) and other

Figure 220 Mast cell naevus in a six month old child to the right of an angioma on the back.

Figure 221 A lesion of mastocytosis has become oedematous and surrounded by erythema after rubbing.

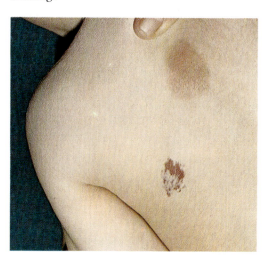

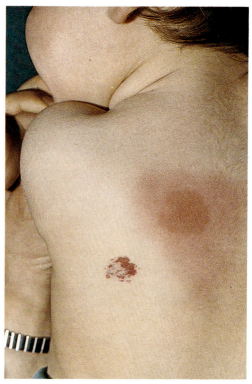

systemic symptoms. Mast cell infiltration may occur in other organs – especially the bones – but generally this has no clinical significance. Very rarely, and usually in the adult, a mast cell leukaemia can occur.

The differential diagnosis includes juvenile xanthogranuloma, but the lesions never urticate in this disease.

Natural history   Typically the lesions become less evident after the first year of life and mostly the disorder has disappeared by the age of six years.

Figure 222 Blister on mast cell naevus on a child of nine months old.

Figure 223 Maculopapular mastocytosis in a one year old child. Note the brownish colour of the lesions.

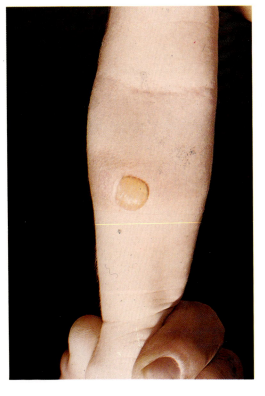
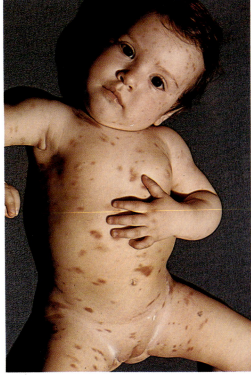

Treatment Usually no treatment is required but if the generalized effects of histamine are troublesome, antihistamines may be used. It is important that histamine-liberating drugs are not given to children with the disease. Aspirin, for example, has caused severe reactions from the sudden release of histamine into the circulation.

Figure 224 Papules of masto-cytosis in a child of eleven months. Many lesions are urticarial and there is a facial flush from liberations of histamine.

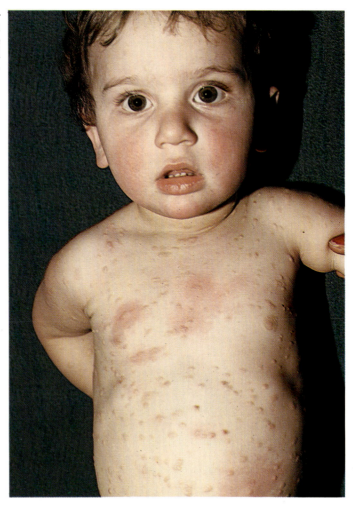

Juvenile xanthogranuloma

This disorder is due to proliferation of histiocytic cells which become lipidized before finally resolving spontaneously – as with many other lesions characterized by cell proliferation in the early years of life (for example, angioma and mastocytosis). The lesions are multiple (Figure 225) or solitary (Figure 226) and start in the first few months of life as small papules or nodules. They later become yellowish and eventually resolve, leaving mild atrophy. It is rare for other organs to be involved – but the eye is occasionally affected. There are no accompanying abnormalities of lipid metabolism and the lipid accumulation in histiocytes is due to an abnormality of these cells.

Differential diagnosis Histiocytosis X must be differentiated as these lesions can be yellowish. However, in the form of the disorder known as Letterer-Siwe disease, haemorrhagic papular lesions occur in the seborr–

Figure 225 Isolated yellowish juvenile xanthogranuloma of deltoid region.

Figure 226 Juvenile xanthogranuloma. Small yellowish papular lesions of the face.

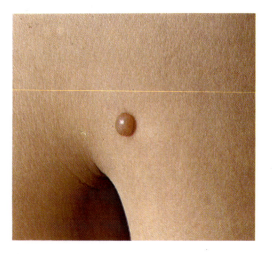

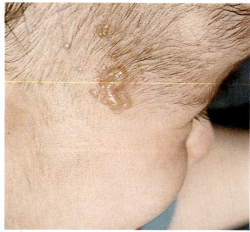

hoeic sites and lesions occur in many viscera. The lesions of mastocytosis may also appear yellowish and be mistaken for xanthogranuloma. However, the lesions of mastocytosis can usually be identified because of their urticating response after stimulation.

One form of the disease occurs on the face (benign cephalic histiocytosis) and adjoining areas alone, so that it is confused with plane warts. This also tends to regress after a few years.

Treatment No treatment is required as the lesions spontaneously resolve.

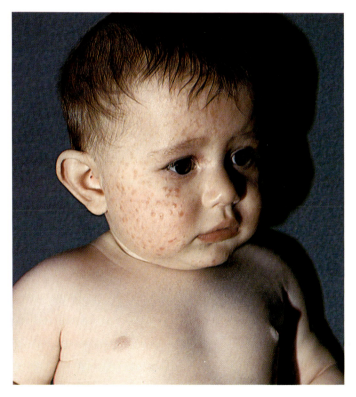

Figure 227 Benign cephalic histiocytosis of the face. Multiple yellowish papular lesions on the face.

Calcifying epithelioma of Malherbe (pilomatrixoma)

Epithelial tumours of the skin are rare in childhood if one excludes xeroderma pigmentosum. This latter is genetically determined and is due to a failure of normal cellular (nuclear DNA) repair mechanisms following solar damage. Malignant skin tumours develop on exposed areas.

The most frequently occurring epithelial tumour of the skin in childhood is the calcifying epithelioma. Generally it occurs on the face and is a rose of whitish-yellow colour (Figure 229). It often has an irregular

Figure 228 Xeroderma pigmentosum. Multiple skin tumours of the face in a child of six.

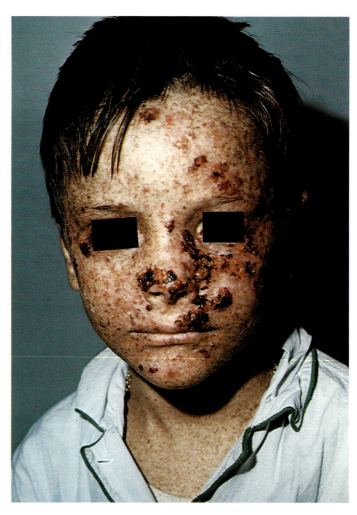

surface and feels quite hard. Histologically it consists of basaloid cells and calcified masses in which are the 'ghosts' of degenerate epidermal cells.

Treatment   Removal, if they are disfiguring, even though they are quite benign.

Figure 229 Calcifying epithelioma of Malherbe. Large lesions of the eyebrows in a child of nine.

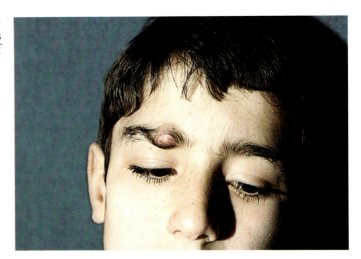

Acknowledgments

We are most grateful to Mrs Hilary Marks for her careful translation from the original Italian and to Professor Ronnie Marks who read the book and made valuable suggestions and corrections.

We have greatly appreciated the help from Roche-Italy in the preparation of the original Italian book.

Finally, we wish to express our gratitude to the publishers for their efficient cooperation.

1986   C.L. MENEGHINI AND E. BONIFAZI

The publishers would like to thank Professor Ronald Marks for supplying the photographs used in Figures 85 and 194, and the Department of Illustration and Teaching Services, Westminster Hospital, London SW1 for Figures 66 and 204.

We are also grateful to Jennifer Eaton, BSc, MSc, MPS for compiling the international drug trade-name table.

International drug trade-name table

UNITED KINGDOM		UNITED STATES	
Generic name	Trade name	Generic name	Trade name
acyclovir	Zovirax	acyclovir	Zovirax
aminocaproic acid	Epsikapron	aminocaproic acid	Amicar
amphotericin	Fungilin	amphotericin B	Fungizone
amphotericin B see amphotericin			

ampicillin	Penbritin; Amfipen;
	  Vidopen; etc.
		ampicillin	Amcill; Omnipen;
			  Totacillin; etc.

aspirin	Solprin; Caprin;
	  Levius; etc.
		aspirin	Ecotrin; Empirin;
			  Bufferin; etc.

benzathine
  penicillin
	Penidural	penicillin G
		  benzathine
			Bicillin

benzyl benzoate
  (lotion)
	Ascabiol	benzyl benzoate
		  (lotion)
			not available

chloroquine	Avloclor; Nivaquine	chloroquine	Aralen
chlortetracycline	Aureomycin	chlortetracycline	Aureomycin
cimetidine	Tagamet	cimetidine	Tagamet
clotrimazole	Canesten	clotrimazole	Lotrimin; Mycelex

disodium cromo-
  glycate see sodium
  cromoglycate			

econazole	Ecostatin; Pevaryl	econazole	Spectazole

epsilon amino
  caproic acid – see
  aminocaproic acid			

erythromycin	Erycen; Erythromid;
	  Ilotycin; etc.
		erythromycin	Eryc; Erythrocin;
			  E-Mycin; etc.

flucytosine	Alcobon	flucytosine	Ancobon
5-fluorocytosine see flucytosine			
5-fluorouracil	Efudix	fluorouracil	Efudex; Fluoroplex
fusidic acid	Fusidin	fusidic acid	not available

gammaglobulin
  see normal
  immunoglobulin			

gammexane see lindane			
griseofulvin	Fulcin; Grisovin	griseofulvin	Fulvicin; Grifulvin; Grisactin

hydrocortisone
  (cream)
	Dioderm; Dome-
	  Cort; Efcortelan;
	  etc.
		hydrocortisone
		  (cream)
			Cort-Dome; Eldecort;
			  Dermacort; etc.

UNITED KINGDOM		UNITED STATES	
Generic name	Trade name	Generic name	Trade name
hydroxychloroquine	Plaguenil	hydroxychloroquine	Plaguenil
ketoconazole	Nizoral	ketoconoazole	Nizoral
lindane (lotion)	Quellada; Lorexane	lindane (lotion)	Scabene
miconazole	Daktarin; Monistat	miconazole	Monistat-Derm; Micatin
natamycin	Pimafucin	natamycin	available only as eye preparations
neomycin	Myciguent	neomycin	Myciguent
normal immuno-globulin	Gammabulin; Kabiglobulin	immune globulin	Gamastan; Gammar; Immuglobin
nystatin	Nystan	nystatin	Mycostatin; Nilstat
povidone-iodine	Betadine	providone-iodine	Betadine; PVP-Iodine
prednisolone	Precorisyl; Deltastab; etc.	prednisolone	Deltasone; Orasone; Meticortoid
ranitidine	Zantac	ranitidine	Zantac
silver sulphadiazine	Flamazine	silver sulfadiazine	Silvadene
sodium cromoglycate	Nalcrom; Intal; Opticrom	cromolyn sodium	Intal; Opticrom; Nasalcrom
sodium stibogluconate	Pentostam	sodium stibogluconate	Pentostam
stibogluconate see sodium stibogluconate			
suphamethoxy-pyridazine	Lederkyn	sulfamethoxy-pyridazine	not available
tolnaftate	Tinaderm	tolnaftate	Aftate; Tinactin
triamcinolone	Kenalog; Lederspan	triamcinolone	Kenalog; Aristospan

Index

collodion film, 46
colon, carcinoma, 12
common warts, 42–4
complex haemangiomas, 30–2
condylomata acuminata, 37, 42–5
congenital disorders: epidermolysis bullosa, 4; hairy naevus, 7; hypothyroidism, 37; ichthyoses, 3; melanocytic naevus, 6–10, 16; syphilis, 37–9, 94, 95
connective tissue disorders, 153–6
corns, 43
corticosteroids: for alopecia areata, 144, 145, 146; for anaphylactoid purpura, 131; for atopic dermatitis, 116–17; for connective tissue disorders, 153, 155, 156; for cutaneolaryngeal angiomatosis, 32; for drug hypersensitivity, 34; for hepatic angioma, 31; and napkin dermatitis, 93–4, 97; for nodular scabies, 82; for psoriasis, 141–2; for seborrhoeic dermatitis, 136–7; for sweat rashes, 88; for vitiligo, 149
Coxsackie virus infections, 40–1, 62
cryotherapy, wart removal, 45
curettage, warts, 45
Cushing's syndrome, 97
cutaneo-laryngeal angiomatosis, 31, 32
cutaneous leishmaniasis, 74–5
cutaneous vasculitis, 59

dapsone, 152
dermatitis: allergic contact, 108, 111, 120; dermatitis artefacta, 98–9; dermatitis herpetiformis, 150–2; factitial, 98–9; irritant contact, 90; napkin, 66, 89–97, 109, 133, 138, 139; photodermatitis, 87; seborrhoeic, 95, 108, 109, 114, 132–7; see also atopic dermatitis
dermatomyositis, 153, 154–5
dermatophagoides, 76
dermatophyte infections, 66, 67, 70–1, 93
dermographic urticaria, 126
dermographism, 101–2
diabetes, 72, 148, 156
diaminodiphenylsulphone, 152
diarrhoea, 92, 94
dichromates, allergic contact dermatitis, 108
diet: and atopic dermatitis, 102, 104, 116; and urticaria, 125–7
discoid lupus erythematosus, 153
disodium cromoglycate, 115
disseminated intravascular coagulation (DIC), 20, 25, 31
dithranol, 142

DNCB, 145
dogs: microsporum canis, 67; ticks, 83
drug reactions, 34–5; erythema multiforme, 63; fixed drug eruption, 40, 60–2, 124, 128–9; napkin dermatitis, 92
dyshidiotic eczema, 35
dyspnoea, 32

echo virus, 62
econazole, 67, 97
eczematization, scabies, 79, 82
electrocoagulation, spider naevi, 29
encephalitis, 83, 108
ephelides, 12
epidermal naevus, 8–10, 16
epidermolysis bullosa, 4–5
epidermolysis bullosa dystrophica, 4–5
epidermolysis bullosa simplex, 4
epinephrine, 127
ipithelial tumours, 162–3
epsilon amino caproic acid, 127
erysipelas, 36
erythema nodosum, 63
erythema multiforme, 63, 65
erythromycin, 35, 115
excoriated acne, 98, 99
eyes: haemangioma, 24–5, 26; herpes simplex, 55

factitial dermatitis, 98–9
faeces, napkin dermatitis, 89–90, 96
favus, 70–1
feet, allergic contact dermatitis, 120
filiform warts, 42, 43
5-deoxyuridine, 55
5-fluorocytosine, 73
5-fluorouracil, 46
5-methoxypsoralen, 87
fixed drug eruption, 40, 60–2, 124, 128–9
flat haemangiomas, 19
folliculitis, 33, 35, 48
food allergies, 102, 116, 125–7
freckles, 12
FTA/1gM195 test, syphilis, 39
fungus infections, 66

gammaglobulin, 115
gammexane lotions, 81
gastrointestinal disorders, gluten enteropathy, 152
gastrointestinal parasites, 126
genetic disorders: atopic dermatitis, 100–1; psoriasis, 138

lymphadenopathy, 57, 60
lymphangitis,78
lymphocytes, 101, 113, 114
lymphoproliferative disorders, 72

macular mastocytosis, 157, 158
macules, pityriasis rosea, 58
malabsorption syndrome, 151–2
malignant melanoma, 7, 10, 15
malignant neoplasms, 17
malignant schwannoma, 11
mast cell leukaemia, 158
mast cell naevus, 157, 158
mast cells, 157–8
mastocytosis, 81, 157–9, 160, 161
measles, 60
melanin, 147
melanocytic naevus, congenital, 6–10, 16
melanoma, juvenile, 15; malignant, 7, 10, 15
mentholated oily calamine lotion, 85
methaemoglobinaemia, 152
mica scale, 59
miconazole, 67
microsporon infections, 68, 69
microsporum canis, 67
miliaria, 88, suppurative, 35
miliaria crystallina, 88
miliaria profunda, 88
miliaria rubra, 88
milk, and atopic dermatitis, 102, 116
'milk crusts', 133
mites, house dust, 76, 111, 113–14; scabies,
   76–82
molluscum contagiosum, 56
Mongolian spot, 13
monilial paronychia, 36
morphoea, 155–6
mosquitos, 85
multiple cutaneous angiomata, 31

naevus flammeus (port wine stain), 29, 31
naevus sebaceous, 17
naevus spilus, 8
nails: bacterial paronychia, 36; chronic mucocutaneous candidiasis, 73
napkin dermatitis, 66, 89–97, 109, 133, 138,
   139
napkin psoriasis, 138
natamycin, 114
neck, smooth haemangioma, 28
neomycin, 108, 118, 120
neonatal pemphigus, 150
nickel allergic contact dermatitis, 108, 120

nodular leishmanisasis, 74
non-accidental injuries, 99
non-steroidal anti-inflammatory agents, 61, 63
Norwegian scabies, 79–80
nystatin, 73, 97

oedema: burns, 86; papular urticaria, 85
oesophagus, epidermolysis bullosa, 5
oil of bergamot, 87
oily calamine lotion, 82, 85
onychomycosis, 73
ophiasiform alopecia, 145
oral thrush, 72, 73, 96
osteochondritis, 37, 38

pallor, atopic dermatitis, 101, 102
palmar-plantar lesions, 37
palpebral angioma, 25
palpebral papular urticaria, 85
papilloma viruses, 83, 108
papillomatosis, 12
papova virus, 42, 43
papular mastocytosis, 157, 159
papular urticaria, 35, 76, 77, 81, 84–5, 104, 110
papules, syphilitic, 37, 38
papulovesicles: herpes simplex, 53, 54; scabies,
   77
paraphenylenediamines, 108, 111, 120
parasites, 76–82, 126
Parrot's pseudoparalysis, 37
paryonchia, bacterial, 36
pediculosis capitis, 35, 70
pemphigoid, 152
pemphigus, 150
penicillin, 35, 37, 39
penis, warts, 43
Peutz-Jeghers syndrome, 12
phenylketonuria, 108
phenytoin, 5
phlebotomus papatasii, 74
phosphocreatine kinase, 155
photoallergy, 87
photochemotherapy, 59, 141, 149
photodermatitis, 87
photosensitizing psoralens (PUVA), 141
phototoxicity, 87
physiological saline, 97
pigmentation, vitiligo, 147–9
pilomatrixoma, 162–3
pityriasis alba, 121, 122
pityriasis lichenoides, 59
pityriasis rosea, 58, 59
pityriasis simplex, 121

pityrosporon ovale, 66, 67
placebos, wart removal, 46
plane warts, 42–3, 161
plantar skin, 21
plantar syphiloderma, 38
plantar warts, 42, 43
plastic pants, napkin dermatitis, 96
podophyllin, 46
port wine stain, 29, 31
povidone-iodine, 35, 48, 136
prednisone, 5, 26, 71, 146
pregnancy: herpes gestationis, 150; screening
    for syphilis, 37; spider naevi, 29
prurigo, 76
pruritus, 108
pseudoparalysis, 37, 38
psoralens, 59, 141, 149
psoriasis, 136, 138–42
psychosomatic factors, alopecia areata, 143
pustular psoriasis, 139, 141
pustules, herpes simplex, 53, 54
PUVA (photochemotherapy), 59, 141, 149
pyoderma, superficial, 5, 33–6
pyogenic cocci, 34
pyogenic granuloma, 15
pyramidone, 129
pyrazolidine, 129
pyrexia, 126

radiotherapy, haemangioma, 25–6
raised haemangiomas, 19–27
ranitidine, 115
rashes, viral, 60–2
RAST test (radio-allergosorbent test), 110–11
respiratory tract infections, 126, 131
retinoic acid, 3
rheumatoid arthritis, 153, 156
rheumatoid nodules, 156
rhinitis, 37, 95, 100, 109
ringworm of the body, 67
ringworm of the scalp, 68–71
roseola, 60, 62

Sabouraud's agar, 66
salicylates, 126, 127
salicylic acid, 3, 46, 56, 142
salmon patches, 19, 28
sandfly, 74
sarcoptes scabiei, 76
scabies, 35, 76–82, 104, 110
scalded skin syndrome, 34–5
scaling: atopic dermatitis, 105, 107; ichthyoses,

3; psoriasis, 138
scalp: dermatophyte infections, 67, 70–1; favus,
    70–1; ringworm, 68–71; seborrhoeic
    dermatitis, 132–5; sweat gland abscesses,
    35
scarletiniform rashes, 61, 62
schwannoma, 11
sclerema, 153
scleroderma, 153, 155
sclerosants, 26
scrotal tongue, 124
sebaceous glands, 17, 101
sebaceous naevus, 17
seborrhoeic dermatitis, 95, 108, 109, 114, 132–7
seborrhoeic glands, 132
sebum, 70
selenium sulfide shampoo, 69
shingles, 49–50
silver nitrate, 86
silver sulferdiazine, 5, 86
skin atrophy, 97, 145, 146
smooth haemangiomas, 28–9
sodium cromoglycate, 116
spider naevi, 28–9
Spitz naevus, 15
staphylococcal scalded skin syndrome, 34–5
staphylococcus, 90, 115
staphylococcus aureus, 33, 34
steroid sulphatase deficiency, 3
steroids: for alopecia areata, 146; for
    epidermolysis bullosa, 5; for erythema
    multiforme, 63; treatment of haemangioma,
    26; for urticaria, 127; for vitiligo, 148
stilbogluconate, 75
strawberry naevi, 19
streptococcal infections, 131
stridor, 32
Sturge-Weber syndrome, 30–1
sudamina, 88
sulfonamides, 63, 108, 118, 120, 129
sulfur, 81
sulphaemoglobinaemia, 152
sulphamethoxypyridazine, 128
superficial pyoderma, 5, 33–6
suppressor lymphocytes, 101, 113, 114
suppurative miliaria, 35
Sutton's naevus, 14
sweat glands, 88, 101; abscesses, 35
sweat rashes, 88, 96
sweating, and atopic dermatitis, 118
syphilis, 37–9, 94, 95
syphilitic pemphigus, 37
systemic lupus erythematosus, 153

171

T-lymphocyte suppressor cells, 101, 113, 114
tar preparations, 118, 142, 156
tartrazine, 127
telangiectasia, 19
thallium, 69
thrush, oral, 72, 73, 96
thymopoietin pentapeptide (TP5), 55, 114
tick bites, 83
tics, 98
tinea capitis, 66, 67, 68–9, 145
tolnaftate, 67
tongue: blackberry, 124; geographic, 122–4; scrotal, 124
toxic epidermal necrolysis, 34
transfer factor, 55, 114
triamcinolone, 117
trichophyton fungi, 68
trichotillomania, 68, 98–9, 145
tumours, epithelial, 162–3

ulceration, haemangioma, 24
ultraviolet light: diagnosis of ringworm, 68; photodermatitis, 87; treatment with (UVA), 59, 142
urine, napkin dermatitis, 89–90, 96
urticaria, 102, 103, 104, 125–7; papular, 84–5, 104, 110; pigmentosa, 157–9

vaccination, herpes simplex, 55
vaccinia virus, 108

varicella, 47–8
varicella zoster virus (VZV), 47, 49
varicelliform parapsoriasis, 59
vascular lakes, 25
vasculitis, 63, 130–1, 154
VDRL test, syphilis, 39
venereal disease, 37–9, 43
verrucae vulgares, 42–4
vesiculation, atopic dermatitis, 105, 106
viral eruptions, 60–2
virus infections: and atopic dermatitis, 108; Coxsackie, 40–1, 62; erythema multiforme, 63; herpes, 47–55; warts, 42
vitiligo, 14, 147–9
von Recklinghausen's disease, 8

warts, 42–6, 56, 83, 108, 161
warty epidermal naevus, 8–10, 16
weals, urticaria, 125, 126
Wiskott-Aldrich syndrome, 108
Wood's light, 68

X-rays, 69
xanthogranuloma, 15, 158, 160–1
xeroderma, 3
xeroderma pigmentosum, 162

zinc cream, 97
zinc metabolism, 94